Birthrate Plus

*A Framework for Workforce Planning and
Decision Making for Midwifery Services*

Jean A. Ball

MSc, Dip N (Dist), RGN, RM

and

Marie Washbrook

Dip QA, RGN, RM

Books for Midwives Press
An imprint of Hochland & Hochland Ltd

1898507414

Published by Books for Midwives Press, 174a Ashley Road, Hale, Cheshire, WA15 9SF, England.

First edition

ISBN 1-898507-41-4

British Library Cataloguing in Publication Data
A catalogue record for this book is available from the British Library

Printed in Great Britain by The Cromwell Press

Contents

Foreword

'Changing Childbirth' and the movement towards evidence based care have created a need for fundamental change in the maternity services. Changes in the pattern of care to provide for greater continuity and more women centred rather than institution centred service is crucial to reform of maternity care. In addition, professionals are required to base the decisions they make on information which arises from good evidence.

Over many years Jean Ball and Marie Washbrook have been collecting and analysing data on midwifery work activity systematically and comprehensively. This evidence, and the definition of clear categories for workload estimation, leading to clear formula for estimating appropriate staff levels, is provided in this new book.

The provision of safe staffing levels is fundamental to the safe and sensitive care required of any maternity service, and to changing the pattern of care in line with the recommendations of 'Changing Childbirth'. Moreover the midwifery staffing budget is the largest component of the costs of the maternity services. Managers, therefore, need a scientific method for calculating staff requirements. This book provides such a scientific method and helps managers relate calculations to individual situations.

Birthrate Plus is an essential tool to any manager of midwifery, both in estimating staffing levels reliably, and in making a sound case if costs are to be cut at any cost. This evidence based, but extremely practical book, will be priceless to the midwife managers, those 'linch pins' of secure and sensitive midwifery care. *Birthrate Plus* will help provide good information to control staffing levels, and to convince others of the numbers of staff required.

Start on Birthrate Plus now, it is bound to be one of your most effective activities!

Lesley Page

The Queens Charlotte's Professor of Midwifery Practice
The Centre for Midwifery Practice
Thames Valley University, London and The Hammersmith Hospitals Trust

Acknowledgements

We wish to acknowledge many people who have contributed to the production and preparation of this book.

First the many midwives and midwifery managers who have been involved with us in developing, testing and applying the *Birthrate* system in numerous maternity services and who have been lively and challenging participants in our taught courses.

Special thanks to Shirley Carlton for her patience and skill in putting both the text and data onto word processor, and revising a number of drafts of the book and its calculations.

We also wish to offer our thanks to the *Nuffield Institute for Health, University of Leeds* for permission to use some of the material which was published in the earlier edition of *Birthrate* (copyright J.A Ball and the Nuffield Institute, 1992) and special thanks are due to Professor David Hunter of the Nuffield Institute for Health, for his consistently helpful response to our request for permission.

And last, but never least, to our husbands, Eric and John and our families for their patience, support and encouragement.

Introduction

The purpose of this book is to provide managers of midwifery services with a framework for assessing the numbers of midwives required within a given service. This is based upon the needs of their clients and the way in which the midwifery service is organized, factors which can be extremely variable in different settings.

Determining workforce needs in any health service requires managers to set clear objectives, namely:

- the volume of workload to be met
- the quality of care to be achieved
- the effective and efficient use of resources
- the way in which the organization of the service will enable the objectives to be met.

The volume of workload depends not only on the number of women and their babies who require care each year, but the variety and demand of the personal clinical needs and expectations of those women and their babies.

The clinical and emotional needs of pregnant and parturient women and their babies and families have been described in numerous text books, research reports, consumer group publications and government reports, thus providing a ready basis from which to define and describe the required quality of care to be achieved.

The Report of the House of Commons Select Committee (Winterton, 1992) brought into sharp focus the demand of consumers for more continuity in and control of maternity care.

The recommendations of Winterton, followed by the Report of the Expert Committee on Midwifery (Cumberlege, 1993) brought about major developments in midwifery practice, especially in the community services.

Add to this the demands of a changing management situation, as the internal market system operating within the National Health Service precipitates the need for health service managers to provide accurate costs for their service and to make increasingly difficult decisions about how financial resources should be used. It could be argued that never before have midwifery managers and planners faced such demands for justifying staffing needs, and demonstrating that their decisions are based upon sound, and demonstrable criteria.

We hope that this manual will help to meet this need.

The manual is based upon widespread experience in both research and application of nursing and midwifery workload and workforce planning systems.

Over the last few years we have both been involved in helping a number of maternity services to plan and evaluate workload demands and to produce the most appropriate staffing response. In addition, we have led numerous seminars on the subject and more recently provided, via the Royal College of Midwives, a modular course in workforce planning and decision making for midwifery managers. This has enabled us to learn from and incorporate the experience of numerous midwifery colleagues.

Birthrate

The manual's foundation is the system known as *Birthrate* (Ball, 1988, 1989, 1992) which was developed initially as a measure of intrapartum care staffing needs.

Its score system provides an accurate measure of case-mix as well as providing a basis for assessing midwife staffing needs. In 1994 the Royal College of Obstetricians and Gynaecologists recommended its use in all delivery suites (RCOG, 1994).

Experience in using *Birthrate* in different hospitals showed that the case-mix data also provided a means of determining postnatal care needs in hospital services. However, the bulk of postnatal care lies in the community and the advent of Winterton and Cumberlege led to a variety of different care patterns being developed in different services.

The case-mix produced by *Birthrate* data has been found to be invaluable in assessing workload for community based work, whether based on traditional care patterns or incorporated within caseload based care proposed by Winterton and Cumberlege.

This book seeks to give some clearly defined answers to the question of matching workload and staffing needs. But as the final decision about staffing numbers will also depend upon local factors, clinical policies and patterns of care, it is also designed to inform decision making and option appraisal based upon local needs.

We hope that this book will provide a user-friendly, and (comparatively) easy to follow manual which will enable our colleagues to address these issues for their own service.

What this book is designed to do

This book is meant to be a practical guide and handbook for managers and their colleagues. Readers who wish to address the theoretical arguments underlying the science of nursing or midwifery workforce planning criteria will find other works on the subject listed in numerous references provided in the text.

Full references will also be given at the first mention of a relevant study or report, but in general will not be repeated elsewhere in the text.

How the book is structured

As the book is meant to be a practical guide for managers and others engaged in workforce planning or decision making, we wanted to make it as easy as possible for readers to find the information required to deal with calculating staff needs for particular areas of care. We also wanted, however, to explore within those areas some of the dilemmas and issues which may arise in the real world.

We have therefore divided the book into a number of **units** each of which deals with a particular topic. In each unit, we have divided the information into **sections** which address specific areas of care or issues arising.

In most of the various units we have used real-life examples of *Birthrate* data and local situations which affect workforce planning decisions, and raise a number of questions and options which may face the manager as she/he reviews their staffing needs.

We have used one real-life situation, Cathedral City, to build up a total staffing profile for a typical Maternity Service as the book progresses.

In this way, we hope that we can provide an integrated picture of staffing assessment and the factors which impinge upon decision making, whilst making it 'comparatively' easy to follow the method of assessment in the different situations.

For those who are daunted by figures, we would encourage you to see that the calculations shown are based on fairly simple arithmetic and that as one becomes more confident in interpreting the data, these figures can provide you with invaluable information upon which to demonstrate the basis for your staffing decisions and to review the impact of various options.

UNIT ONE

The Development of Workforce Planning Systems

In this first unit we are setting the scene by exploring some of the concepts and issues which underlay the development of nursing workload and workforce assessment systems, the problems and pitfalls encountered, together with some of the lessons learnt.

Finally we will explore the processes which need to take place if sound decisions are to be made in service or workplace planning debates.

Section 1.1: Reviews the development of nursing workload system in the United Kingdom and the main approaches which emerged. A number of references will indicate areas for further reading on this subject.

Section 1.2: Explores some of the problems and pitfalls which surrounded these developments and the valuable lessons learnt. Many of these were not flattering to either nursing or general managers, but undertaking workload/workforce studies brought to light factors which affect staffing decisions which had not been recognized before these studies were undertaken.

Section 1.3: Discusses the principles of using workload assessments as a component in management decision making in the light of the lessons and offers a model of the processes required for sound service and workforce planning.

Comment

Some midwives become irritated when lessons or models drawn from nursing are used in midwifery situations. I think that this is a sad mistake and is not appropriate in research. The principles and tested methods of assessing patient or client needs of nursing, midwifery or medical care can be applied in different situations *providing that their concepts and descriptions of client need and staff activity has been defined in a way related to the service being assessed (JAB).*

Section 1.1

Concepts and development of workforce planning methods

Introduction

This introduction to the development of workforce planning systems is intended to provide an overview of the various systems which have been developed in the United Kingdom. Further details of these methods can be found in the recommended reading given at the end of this section. Of these the following are particularly recommended:

1.   Hurst, K. (1993). *Nursing Workforce Planning*. Harlow: Longman.

      This invaluable book reviews the details of 80 methods developed from 1976 onwards, analyses the strengths and weaknesses of the main systems and guides the readers in their application.

2.   Ball, J.A. (1993). 'Workload measures in midwifery' in Alexander, J., Levy, V., Roch, S. (Eds). *Midwifery Practice; A Research-Based Approach* Vol. 4, Basingstoke: Macmillan.

Historical background

Throughout the history of health services there has been a pattern of meeting demands for care with the resources available. Thus in the pre-NHS days, hospitals were either voluntary or provided by the local authority. In the voluntary hospitals patients paid for their care (or received help from some charitable fund) and most consultants gave their time free (in addition to their private practice both within and without the hospital). The local authority hospitals provided some acute but mainly chronic and geriatric care together with community nursing and midwifery services.

In all of these hospitals probationer nurses staffed the wards, undertaking most of the domestic and nursing duties 'in return for their training'. They were easily disciplined by the threat of dismissal and formed a cheap labour force.

During the war years, some hospitals employed ward orderlies, some had auxiliary or assistant nurses, later to become state enrolled nurses.

Determining how many nurses was an issue for the Matron of a hospital and the degree to which she could persuade her Hospital Management Committee to fund the staff required. Some community services adopted a more objective method by assessing the number of district nurses, midwives or health visitors per 1000 population.

Coming of the National Health Service

These conditions continued through many of the early years of the NHS, until the 1960s when there began an extensive hospital building programme, with increases in the number and variety of medical consultants, developments in clinical treatments and diagnostic services and changes in the role of student nurses.

Strategic planning needs

The hospital building programme planners began to look for some formula for costing the nursing staff required to match the new developments. Thus all the early approaches to workforce planning were 'top-down' i.e. arising from strategic planning rather than operational needs. This means that they assessed the nursing staff needed to match the planned patterns of care, but were not used to assess the effect of changes in the volume of developments in care.

Notable examples of the strategic planning methods produced include the Scottish Health and Hospital Boards (Aberdeen Formula, 1969) and the Oxford Regional Health Authority (Barr et al, 1967, 1972, 1984), both of which began to address the issue of determining ward workload by assessing patient dependency on nursing care and then calculating the time needed to meet each level of dependency.

The only study which addressed midwifery services was that of Auld (1976) who was then Chief Nursing Officer for Scotland.

None of these studies used any objective method of the quality of care being produced, rather they studied typical wards where it was assumed that the care was of an acceptable standard.

The need for operational measures of nursing workload

The 1980s saw an increasing need for bottom-up methods of assessing nursing requirements. This was driven by a rapidly developing service with attendant costs, changes in the structure of the service after the integration of all health care services under the NHS in 1974 and the lack of any methods for costing services, driven further by the growing financial burden of the health service. Increasingly NHS management at local level needed information upon which to base its decisions.

Issues of quality objectives and targets

It was at this time that questions began to be asked about the quality of care to be achieved. This was an issue first faced by Senior (1979) who attempted to assess the nursing time required for good quality care by ensuring that the wards under review had ample staff during the period of study, and asked each ward sister to assess the quality of care being provided.

Although this was a rather subjective approach it nevertheless raised important issues:

- what are the objectives of care?
- to what standards are these objectives being met?

The need to address quality as part of the workforce planning process was encapsulated in the work of Goldstone and Ball who produced an integrated system published as *Monitor; An Index of the Quality of Nursing Care for Medical and Surgical Wards* (Goldstone and Ball et al., 1983) and a workload assessment methodology *Criteria for Care* (Ball and Goldstone et al., 1984). Ball (1984) suggests that the question to be addressed in any system of workforce planning is:

> 'How many nurses are needed to provide defined standards of care to a defined group of patients?'

Different approaches to workload assessment and workforce planning produced in the 1980s

OBJECTIVE ASSESSMENT METHODS

Broadly the patterns produced two main methods of bottom-up assessment of nursing workload:

1. Standard times for nursing tasks/interventions
   (Auld, 1976; Bell and Storey, 1984).
   This method assessed, either by observation or consensus, the time required to carry out various aspects of nursing care. By relating the number of interventions required by patients in different client/dependency groups, it was possible to calculate the average nursing time required per day or week for a specified group of patients.

2. Dependency based systems
   This method classified patients into various categories of need for nursing care and measured by non-participant observation, the time per day required to meet the needs of each category (Barr et al., 1972; Rhys-Hearn, 1974; Ball et al., 1984). The method developed by Ball et al (1984, 1986; Ball, 1987) incorporated a quality measure and restricted the basis for calculating staff needs by only using the criteria produced by wards which achieved a minimum of 70 per cent of the quality standards listed in *Monitor* (Goldstone and Ball, 1983). Later studies addressed issues of skill mix (Ball et al., 1989; Ball and Hurst, 1990).

Both the standard time and dependency based methods added extra staff time for indirect care and associated work. By applying the times produced to a continuing collection of dependency and/or nursing data for each ward, an ongoing assessment of the staff required by patient workload can be produced.

Two other methods took a different approach:

CONSENSUS METHODS
Telford (1983) produced a profile with which ward sisters assessed their ward activities and produced their conclusions of staff needed for each shift.

CLINICAL INDICATORS IN INTENSIVE CARE UNITS
(Knaus et al., 1981, 1982; Morgan, 1986).
This method, primarily designed as a strategic planning tool, identified clinical criteria of the patients' physical state, gave them scores according to the degree of need, and used these to allocate patients into low, intermediate and high dependency categories. The nursing time required per shift per category was defined respectively as half a nurse, one nurse and two nurses.

A similar approach was taken in *planning* for Special and Intensive Care of the Newborn (British Paediatric Association and Royal College of Obstetricians, 1977, 1982, 1977, 1982; Royal College of Physicians, 1988; British Perinatal Society and the Neonatal Nurses Association, 1992).

Developments in midwifery
Since Auld's (1976) first study of midwifery workload there have been some attempts to assess midwifery workload. Maclean and Bowden (1988) described the initial results of a standard time approach to assessing workload in postnatal care.

Birthrate (Ball, 1988, 1992) uses the *clinical indicator* approach to allocate clients into various categories of need for intrapartum care together with measures of midwife time needed to meet the needs of various categories. Further work (Ball et al., 1992) uses something of the *consensus/standard time* approach, as do other developments, in assessing staff for hospital wards and departments and community based care. All of these will be addressed in this manual.

Section 1.2

Problems, pitfalls and lessons learnt during the development and application of nursing workforce systems

A number of valuable lessons have been learnt from the experience of developing, applying and interpreting the results of nursing workload/workforce planning systems.

Problems and pitfalls

In the early days, an assumption was made that a workload system alone could provide the answers to staffing issues. As a result there was much criticism and arrogance about different methods of measurement, often because the users did not like the results obtained. But workload/workforce data simply produces an important component in the decision making process. In 'good' situations where there was a healthy research based approach such questions led to further study, debate, evaluation and learning.

Lessons learnt

ISSUES OF METHODOLOGY

All methods have their strengths, weakness and limitations and these should be understood in the context of overall decision making.

Any method used to assess workload should have a clearly defined link to standards of quality, service targets and objectives. If this is done, then the implication of the data for care management can be readily assessed and different options or solutions can be produced.

Methods used should be capable of demonstrating changes in the volume and intensity of workload demands over time. This is usually achieved when the data provides a detailed case-mix for different client groups or care settings.

Unless data is used, collecting it is an expensive and demotivating exercise. Also the time spent and costs of collecting data should be measured against the usefulness of the data for workload control, staffing decisions and quality evaluation.

The results should form one component in the decision making process which includes assessing performance against objectives, cost-effectiveness, forward planning etc.

HOW THE RESULTS WERE RECEIVED

Unfortunately, the development of workload planning systems also exposed the fact that:

- many managers found it difficult to understand and apply the information gained (see Audit Commission Reports, 1991, 1992)

- there is a dearth of numeracy skills at all levels in the NHS.

VALUABLE INSIGHTS GAINED

On a more positive note, where data were correctly used and issues addressed then these valuable lessons were learned:

- the context in which a service is provided makes a difference to the use of workforce planning data

- unplanned changes in workload volume or case-mix produces serious effects upon nursing time available, patient care and quality issues

- some wards/specialities have potential for using their nursing resources more flexibly than others (Ball and Oreschnik, 1986; Ball, 1987; Ball et al., 1989; Ball and Hurst, 1989)

- professional and managerial expertise and judgement plays a vital role in using workload data correctly as part of the management process

- the continuing use of workforce planning systems, *Criteria for Care* and *Birthrate*, demonstrated that robust data built up over time can provide a framework for successfully predicting workload/workforce demands based upon planned or expected changes (Ball and Hurst, 1989).

Section 1.3

Principles of workload assessment as a component of management decision making

As a result of the increased understanding of workload measurement outlined previously and of our continuing experience in working with midwifery and general managers, the following concepts/model of the workforce planning scenario is proposed. All of the factors described play a significant role in determining the workforce required to match the needs of clients of a health service, and must be addressed if sound decisions are to be made.

Measuring the demand for care

- In determining the method of workload assessment to be used, it is more valid to focus on the *needs of the client* than upon the *activities of nurses/midwives*. This is because the *activities* of staff may or may not be appropriate to the client's needs or may not produce the most efficient use of resources.

  For example, many wards in the first *Criteria for Care* studies were providing less than 70 per cent of the required care, despite lots of activity (Ball et al., 1986, 87). In other studies, staff were spending a large percentage of their time in non-nursing activities (Gillett and Flux, 1987; Ball et al., 1989) and there was considerable evidence that they would be reluctant to relinquish many of these non-nursing duties (Ball et al., 1989).

  Focusing on activity encourages the continuance of the status quo.

- Assessing resources should always be related to defined objectives of care/ service and to quality standards required within the particular service. In midwifery we have numerous reports, guidelines etc. which all define desired standards of care.

- Data should be easy to collect and understandable. It should be easy to check the reliability of data and its resulting calculations.

Effect of context, geography of area under review and reality factors

A number of issues have been found which affect or add to the staffing requirements produced by workforce planning methods. These are defined as the geography of the area under review and include the following:

- size of wards/units
- distances covered by community services
- patterns of care, clinical policies, restraints, duty of care issues

- work allocation and shift patterns
- degrees of potential for flexibility in working patterns.

Where any of these factors are not open to change we have defined them as *reality factors*.

Professional judgement and management skill

There has been a tendency to dismiss professional judgement as 'subjective' and therefore dubious or as irrelevant. Certainly workload data should be as objective as possible and be presented in a form that is understandable to all managers. But professional judgement based on experience is a vital component in the *interpretation and application* of results.

Similarly management skill in allocating priorities, determining objectives and targets to be met is crucial if planning of services is to be both effective and efficient.

Processes required for sound service/workforce planning

The model shown below attempts to show how these various components fit together in forming a robust and sensitive workforce/service planning system.

1.	Assessing the demand:
a)	client needs and quality targets produces assessment of resources of time and skill needed to provide required level of service.
	↓
b)	Results tempered by: appraisal of quality issues - any changes needed? geography factors - additions, restraints, variations needed initial staffing options - numbers, skill mix produced.
	↓
2.	Professional judgement used:
a)	to assess quality, geography issues marked as above and to produce solutions to issues raised, including appraisal of the strengths and weaknesses of different options.
b)	further refinement of staffing options: numbers, skill mix, deployment.
	↓
3.	Management decisions made in light of 1 and 2 and in relation to unit wide priorities, demands, targets and constraints.
	↓
4.	Final staffing numbers agreed for defined period of time. Decisions published in the context of care objectives to be met.
	↓
5.	Plans made for review and reassessment.

Fig. 1.1: Components and processes needed to achieve sound workforce/service planning

UNIT TWO

How Birthrate was Developed as a Method for Assessing Client Need for Midwifery Care during Intrapartum Care

In this unit, we will explain how Birthrate developed: the basic principles of the system, how it was developed and piloted and its further application to other areas of midwifery care.

Introduction and acknowledgements

Section 2.1: Discusses how *Birthrate* was developed as a measure for staffing intrapartum care and the basic principles upon which the system is based.

Section 2.2: Explains the basic principles upon which *Birthrate* is based and how the chosen method was tested.

Section 2.3: Outlines the further testing of Birthrate system in seven hospitals and how its data can help in informing decisions about other areas of care.

Introduction

Birthrate: its history, basic principles and developments
History of the development of Birthrate

The work which led up to the development of *Birthrate* began in North Lincolnshire Health District in 1985. It began as a joint venture based upon the mutual interest of Jean Ball (then Senior Nurse Research at the District Headquarters), and the labour ward midwives at Lincoln County Hospital.

It may be important to point out that, apart from the important resource of staff time, no specific funding was available for developing a midwifery workforce planning system, although later validation of the Birthrate tool was undertaken as part of the Trent Regional Health Authority Project (Trent Health, 1991).

Due acknowledgement and many thanks are due to the countless midwives who have contributed to the work over the years.

In 1992 funds were provided by the Department of Health Resource Management Project which paid part of the costs of publishing *Birthrate* via the Nuffield Institute at the University of Leeds (Ball, 1992).

Section 2.1

Setting the foundations for the development of Birthrate

Intrapartum care as basis for the system

The major objective of maternity care is to ensure the safe delivery of a healthy baby wherever possible.

An early decision was to concentrate the development within intrapartum care as this was regarded as the fulcrum around which all other maternity care revolves. Antenatal care is designed to identify any potential problems well before the onset of labour, and the pattern of postnatal is affected by the outcome of labour for mother and baby.

Therefore, if we could classify women and their babies in terms of their need for midwife care during labour, the resulting data should help us to identify postnatal care needs as well.

Research dilemmas

However choosing intrapartum care as the basis for measuring workload raised a number of other problems. High fluctuation of numbers and unpredictability of the processes of labour and delivery meant that normal approaches to measuring staff time and activity would be difficult because:

- the unpredictability of intrapartum care meant that there could be a danger of measuring staff inputs at time when the staff available did not match client need.
- the workload in a delivery suite can vary greatly from day to day and crises can occur at any time.
- the admission of patients to a delivery suite (apart from elective caesareans) is not controllable. Labour and delivery inevitably follow 40 or more weeks of pregnancy at any time of day or night.

Attempting to measure staff activity would mean extensive observation over a long period of time in order to gain any notion of 'patterns' of care, and would be prohibitively expensive, and might not provide the most useable type of information.

Activity analysis is only useful as an aid to workforce planning if the workload can be controlled, restricted or rescheduled, which is not the case in intrapartum care.

However, there were some advantages in studying intrapartum care:

A. USING PATIENT EPISODES AS A BASIS FOR ASSESSMENT
Although bed occupancy was not a relevant measure of workload demand, the fact that the vast majority of clients stay in the delivery suite for less than 24 hours meant

that an assessment using single patient episode could be used as basic component of workload assessment.

B. DIRECT CARE IS THE MAJOR COMPONENT OF THE WORK

As previous government reports had defined the desired standard of midwife attendance on a woman in labour to be '*the undivided attention of a midwife throughout labour and delivery*' (Short Report, 1980; Maternity Services Advisory Committee Report on Intrapartum Care, 1985), then it would be comparatively easy to measure the basic input of midwife time per client by measuring the time between admission in labour to transfer out of the delivery suite after the birth.

For all these reasons, it was decided to seek a means of classifying women according to their need of care during the processes of labour and delivery and to include a measure of the health of the newborn infant.

This raised the major research question, *how to classify mothers and babies in a way which reflected midwife workload and client need?*

Addressing the research issues

There were a number of problems to be considered in producing a valid means of classifying client needs in a way which reflected the variability of events in labour and delivery, and the amount of midwifery input needed to provide appropriate levels of care.

The usual outcome measure for intrapartum care was to record the number of complicated deliveries e.g. forceps, breech, caesarean, etc. together with details of stillbirths, neonatal deaths, premature and small for dates babies. However, these outcomes did not provide a sound basis for assessing midwifery workload, as they reflected only the outcome, rather than the processes which had led to the outcome. Neither did they include the highest percentage of birth outcomes, namely the 'normal delivery'.

Normal delivery is the term used to describe a normal vaginal delivery. However, a *normal delivery* might follow a labour which had required a high degree of intervention e.g. fetal monitoring, diabetic control, or follow a long exhausting labour.

The growing availability of epidural analgesia was another factor which had increased the workload of midwives in an otherwise normal or uncomplicated labour and delivery. Add to this the possibility of complications for the infant, retained placenta or postpartum haemorrhage, and the number of variables which might be involved in a 'normal vaginal delivery' seemed to be limitless.

Similarly, an emergency caesarean section might follow hours of labour or a failed forceps delivery or might involve twins, all of which require a high input of midwifery and obstetric time and skill.

It was therefore decided that we needed to produce a tool which could identify key indicators of need, and yet be relatively easy to complete after the birth of the baby.

Section 2.2

Basic principles, developing and testing the system

It is important to understand that the basic principle of the system is to focus *on the client's needs rather than midwife activity* as the measure of required time.

> *Comment:* I had planned to use the term basic to describe the 'bottom-line' standards of care, staff numbers etc. However it seems that although the word basic means 'constituting a basis, underlying, simple with no extras' (Universal Dictionary, 1986), it has of late become almost synonymous with 'sparse, of poor quality, the least we can get away with'. Therefore I have decided to use the term *fundamental* to describe the starting point from which all other measures, concepts and decisions arise (JAB).

Defining the needs of the clients

It was decided to base the system on the clinical indicator approach used in intensive care units (Knaus et al., 1981, 1982).

The assessment would be a retrospective assessment of need based on events of labour and delivery. This would allow for all eventualities and not interfere with care delivery.

It would be easy to cross-check with records for validity and reliability. Details of the clinical indicators can be seen on the score sheet.

What is the quality standard?

The quality standard was already defined as one midwife to one mother throughout labour (Short, 1980; MSAC, 1985). Therefore the length of time a woman spent in labour should be the fundamental standard of midwife time input. However some situations and certain clinical policies require more than one midwife to be in attendance, and this also needed to be taken into consideration.

How will midwife time be measured?

The fundamental measurement would be the total time that the woman required the care of a midwife/midwives, either in the hospital, in the woman's home or in the case of domino deliveries, a combination of the two. In the light of later development of caseload based working, this proved to be a very helpful decision.

The volume of midwife time needed would be increased when certain interventions, events or crises intervened and it was decided to assess this need via the clinical indicator system. Experience in some units also taught that it is crucial to include time spent by a woman in labour and cared for on an antenatal ward before being transferred to delivery suite.

Other workload in delivery suites

Undertaking the research revealed other work in delivery suites which needed to be recorded:

1.   Women admitted but not delivered:
        Category X - false alarms
        Category A - women needing antenatal care/interventions

2.   Women re-admitted after delivery mainly for surgery:
        Category R - repair of trauma, tubal ligations, etc.

3.   Midwives from delivery suite undertaking escort duties, flying squad calls or attending women in operating theatres in another area of the hospital.

Development and piloting of system

Clinical indicators were derived from:

•   normal obstetric and midwifery practice
•   midwives' identification of issues/events which added to their workload e.g. maintaining epidural analgesia, caesarean sections.

Once the indicators were identified, scores were allocated according to the degree of severity or potential need for increased support. The method was drawn from qualitative research techniques and the intensive care scores (Knaus et al, 1981) e.g. 35 week gestation with normal process but increased need to monitor health of fetus, support anxious parents.

By adding the scores it was hoped to classify mothers and babies into a number of dependency groups. The fundamental group, Group I, would reflect the perfectly normal labour and delivery where the gestation was 37 weeks or more, length of labour was eight hours or less, normal delivery, intact perineum, infant with apgar score of eight or more at five minutes, birth weight more than 2.5 kgms.

Validation

Once the score system was set up a trial run of six months data was undertaken. The validity of the scores was then checked by blind checking of the records for the same six months. This work was undertaken by an independent researcher who had not been involved with any of the foregoing development.

First, all the cases which would normally have been considered complicated and were recorded in the delivery suite review book e.g. forceps delivery, elective and emergency caesareans, diabetic mother, babies needed resuscitation, stillbirths etc. were compared against the score sheet completed at the time of delivery. Then the other cases classed as vaginal deliveries were also compared.

The results are as shown in the following table:

Classification Groups	Vaginal deliveries		Elective caesarean section		Emergency caesarean section		TOTAL	
	No.	%	No.	%	No.	%	No.	%
Group I	204	100	nil		nil		204	100
Group II	607	100	nil		nil		607	100
Group III	161	100	nil		nil		161	100
Group IV	152	92.7	12	7.3	nil		164	100
Group V	45	35.2	36	28.1	47	36.7	128	100
TOTALS	1169		48		47		1264	

Table 2.1: Number and percentage of case in each classification group which ended as vaginal deliveries, emergency or elective caesareans

It can be seen that although the caesarean sections come in groups IV and V as might be expected, there are still a large number of vaginal deliveries in these high dependency groups. Further analysis revealed that of the 358 vaginal deliveries in groups III - V:

- 73 per cent of Category III followed a normal labour and delivery plus epidural and longer labour or episiotomy, in short, normal processes with some extra support or intervention; 12 per cent were forceps deliveries plus episiotomy and 8 per cent had a combination of minor variables, longer labour, under 37 weeks gestation with small but healthy baby, etc.

- 78 per cent of Category IV were women with some problem; for example needing induction, continuous fetal monitoring, or having some medical condition such as diabetes, plus epidural, or forceps delivery.

Included in the 45 who fell into Category V were: two sets of twins with normal or forceps deliveries; one stillbirth; several small for dates babies who needed a good deal of help at birth; plus one woman with a heart condition who had an elective forceps under epidural; one with a retained placenta; two with some degree of postpartum haemorrhage; plus other women who needed a number of interventions but who had succeeded in giving birth vaginally with a healthy baby.

These results were later confirmed when other maternity units tested the system, and in seven major maternity units in the Trent Health Region. Analysis of their data did not identify any 'outliers' in terms of the total scores which might indicate situations which had not been allowed for in the basic score system. Further details of the Trent RHA data can be found in 'Workload Measures in Midwifery' (Ball, 1993).

We do not know precisely how many units are using the system at the present time but at least 50 services are known to the authors, suggesting that the score system is valid in any intrapartum service. The recent recommendation of *Birthrate* by the Royal College of Obstetricians (RCOG, 1994) also suggests that the system has been found to be valid.

Reliability checks

All the score sheets produced by the pilot study were checked for correct recording of the time spent by the woman in the delivery suite and 94 per cent were found to be correct. However there were less accuracy in midwives' skill in calculating time, as only 89 per cent had been correct in their arithmetic. However, these are regarded as good reliability results.

Time measurements

The time measurements per classification group or category confirmed the validity of the tool for assessing midwife time. There was a clear sequence of time increase as the clinical indictor score increased. This is interesting in view of the fact that only Group I restricted the length of time in labour to eight hours or less, and the sequential increase in time reflects longer labours, increased intervention at delivery, suturing after delivery etc.

System easy to use

The system was found to be easy to use by midwives, and rapidly became part of the final record keeping chore required for all deliveries.

Summary

The *Birthrate* score system validly reflected the needs of mothers and babies during labour and delivery (and indeed can be use as a quality audit tool - see later discussion).

The retrospective nature of the system made it easy to collect the data at the end of intrapartum care and its completion did not interfere with the care of the woman during labour.

The time measurement could be checked against the time spent by the woman in the delivery suite.

Section 2.3

Further application and uses of the Birthrate data in midwifery workforce assessment

The initial work was completed in Lincoln in 1986, and then tested further in nine hospitals (seven in Trent Health Region) during 1988/89.

Continuing application and research in a number of units showed that the case-mix produced by *Birthrate* could be used to predict and assess workload and workforce needs in other areas.

As the work progressed it was found that the clinical indicator approach accurately predicted client needs for postnatal care. This, combined with clearly defined patterns of midwifery care, enabled assessment of *postnatal* beds (Ball, 1992) and later staffing needs for postnatal wards to be based on the *Birthrate* outcome category for both hospital and community based care.

Measuring midwife activity in wards had the same problems of unpredictability and lack of control as the delivery suite, but patient sample was less prone to variation than those in general hospital wards because:

- normal healthy women whose progress after birth was largely predictable

- where complications had arisen for mother or baby, this had been identified in the *Birthrate* category.

Adding information from other studies

TEAM/CASELOAD BASED MIDWIVES

The advent of the proposals of Winterton (1992) and later Cumberlege (1993) led to other work which explored the development and feasible workload of caseload based midwives and teams or group practices. The experiences and conclusions of these studies (Ball et al, 1992; Wraight et al, 1993; Flint, 1995; Page, 1995) added to assessment of case-mix via *Birthrate*, provided a useful framework for assessing midwife time needed by different patterns of caseload based work for home or hospital births.

SPECIAL NEEDS OF SMALL UNITS

Experience in nursing workload helped us to deal with the problems in using workload based staffing requirements in units with small numbers of deliveries, and in calculating the need for health care assistants etc. (Ball et al, 1989; Audit Commission, 1992 p.38)

A similar approach was taken to assess the staff needed for antenatal clinics and parentcraft classes in hospital services.

TESTING THE METHODS

All these developments came about as the result of application in numerous maternity units of differing size, case-mix and with different permutations of midwifery practice. The experience and understanding gained by this work forms the basis for this book and will be discussed in more detail in the following units of this manual.

UNIT THREE

How to Use the Birthrate System

This unit explains in detail how to use the Birthrate system to calculate workload and staffing needs for intrapartum care.

It demonstrates the kind of data that are produced and how they can be used to calculate workload indices and determine staffing needs.

Further sections explain how to set the system up within a service, how to collate the information and undertake reliability checks.

A number of exercises are included which are designed to give an opportunity to use the system and to make management judgements on the results.

Section 3.1: Explains how to use Birthrate, copyright issues and the score system.

Section 3.2: Provides the instructions on how to complete the score sheet to produce the five categories of need for women who have given birth and a further three categories for other women who may be cared for in the delivery suite.

Section 3.3: Explains how the midwife time needed is determined.

Section 3.4: Provides an exercise in scoring the clinical indicators for several case-studies and assess the length of time in the delivery suite.

Section 3.5: Explains how to set up the system within a maternity unit and how to ensure reliability of data.

Section 3.6: Discusses how to use the Birthrate data to:

      a)   calculate staffing needs for delivered cases
      b)   produce workload ratios and indices
      c)   calculate staffing for other cases, flying squad and escort duties

Section 3.7: Provides a different set of exercises designed to give experience in calculating staff from data and raises a number of other issues:

a)   the effect of different care policies upon staffing needs
b)   working out staffing needs based on the actual Birthrate data of two different sized hospitals

Section 3.8: This final section discusses some of the management issues raised by the data and the results provided in the two sets of exercises.

Summary

Section 3.1

How to use Birthrate
Basic principles

Delivery suites are like intensive care units; they operate an emergency driven service to clients (mothers and babies both before and after birth) which requires high levels of attention and care. At any time during the processes of labour and delivery, emergency intervention may be needed to preserve the life and health of the mother or her baby.

Therefore, as stated in the Short Report (1980), the standard of attention required is at least one midwife to one mother throughout the time the mother is in the delivery suite. In complicated cases, more than one midwife is required for some of this time.

Once this 'quality standard' has been grasped, the *midwife time per case category is sufficient to provide all the direct and indirect care, including all the paperwork,* which is needed to give undivided attention to a mother, her partner and her baby during labour, throughout delivery and in the immediate post birth time on the delivery suite.

Birthrate is a *retrospective assessment* of the events and factors arising in the labour and delivery process, and uses a *score system* based upon *clinical indicators* of the needs of women and their infants.

The score obtained is used to assign the client and her baby to one of five *categories of need*. Three other categories are provided for other clients cared for in a delivery suite.

This method is similar to that used in intensive care units in general hospitals and has been carefully validated. Therefore it is inadvisable to change or add to the score system.

It is important that midwives understand these basic principles and *do not* add 'extra' indicators for particular clients.

Copyright issues

The methods described within this manual may be used freely within maternity services, provided that due acknowledgement is always given to the original source by referencing Ball and Washbrook (1996). Previous copyright was Ball (1992).

The copyright note on the score sheet should be maintained on any copies or other records, including computer based record systems.

The *Birthrate* system provides:

- A score system based upon various clinical indicators for women who have been delivered
- Special categories for women who have not yet been delivered or who have been re-admitted following delivery
- A record of the length of time each woman has spent in the delivery suite
- A method for recording time spent on flying squad, escort duties etc
- A staffing formula.

Principles of classifying maternal and neonatal factors in the process and outcome of labour and delivery

The score sheet is completed at the time that the *mother leaves the delivery suite.*

The purpose of classifying mothers in different groups according to their degree of need for midwifery care is to identify differences among them which would require different degrees of midwifery and medical attention during labour and delivery, and to define a variety of outcomes.

All women in labour require careful monitoring of their physical condition, the process of their labour, accurate assessment of the condition of the fetus and sensitive emotional support. Such aspects of care are regarded as basic for all women. The scoring system is designed to identify and weight these fundamental requirements together with other key indicators of increased needs.

The scoring system provides eight categories for classification. There are five categories for mothers who have given birth during their time in the delivery suite (Categories I-V) and three for other cases (X, A and R).

Details of the first five categories are given below. The other three categories will be described later in this section.

CATEGORY I (SCORE = 6)
This is the most normal and healthy outcome possible. A woman is defined as Category I (lowest level of dependency) if:

- her pregnancy is of 37 weeks gestation or more;
- she is in labour for eight hours or less;
- she achieves a normal delivery with an intact perineum;
- her baby has an Apgar score of 8 + and weighs more than 2.5kg;
- and she does not require or receive any further treatment and/or monitoring.

CATEGORY II (SCORE = 7 - 9)
This is also a normal outcome, very similar to I, but with the addition of induction (score 2) or a perineal tear (2) or a length of labour of more than eight hours (2).

However, if more than one of these events happened, then the mother and baby outcome would be in category III.

CATEGORY III (SCORE = 10 - 13)

In many cases, normal deliveries following epidural and some well managed elective caesarean sections fall into this category.

CATEGORY IV (SCORE = 14 - 18)

More complicated cases affecting mother and/or baby will be in this category, including elective caesarean sections.

CATEGORY V (SCORE = 19 OR MORE)

This score is reached when the mother and/or the baby requires a very high degree of support or intervention. For example, pregnancy is at term, labour lasts 12 hours, the mother has an epidural, delivery is by forceps, and there is a retained placenta, which is removed under general anaesthetic. The mother needs intravenous infusion, and recovers well. The infant's apgar score was less than five at one minute, but then recovered well. All emergency sections and multiple births will fall into Category V.

Changes since the first edition of the score sheet

There have been one or two changes made to the score sheet (Ball, 1992):

1.   In section A:
      Elective anaesthetic has been put here rather than in Section D as before.

2   In the infant section C:
      Paediatrician called at or after delivery has been deleted in the light of developments in intrapartum care.

BIRTHRATE SCORE SHEET

Mother's details	Date of delivery		199
	Length of time in delivery suite		hours

Section A	GESTATION / LABOUR / INTERVENTIONS	
Gestation	37 weeks or more	1
	More than 34 weeks, less than 37	2
	Less than 34 weeks	3
Length of labour	8 Hours or less	1
	More than 8 hours	2
As required	I.V. infusion (*not blood transfusion*)	2
	Epidural in situ	3
	Elective general/spinal anaesthetic	3
	Continuous fetal monitoring	3
*(see note on multiple birth scores)	Twins*	2
	Triplets, quadruplets, etc*	5
	Medical problems needing consultant oversight *e.g. diabetes, heart or chest conditions*	5
	Subtotal SECTION A	

Section B	DELIVERY	
	Normal delivery	1
	Forceps / breech, etc	2
	Elective Caesarean section	3
	Emergency Caesarean section	5
** Must be scored for caesarean section	**Perineum intact	1
	Vaginal/perineal tear/episiotomy	2
	Extended episiotomy/3rd degree tear	3
	Subtotal SECTION B	

Section C	INFANT(S)	
Apgar assessed at 5 minutes	Apgar score 8+	1
	Apgar score between 5 and 7	2
	Apgar score less than 5	3
Multiple births : score each baby	Birth weight 2.5 kg or more	1
	Birth weight 1.5kg - 2.5kg	2
	Birth weight less than 1.5kg	3
As required	Congenital abnormality	3
	Infant is stillborn / dies immediately after birth	5
	Subtotal SECTION C	

Section D	OTHER INTENSIVE CARE	
	I.V. infusion **started or maintained** post-delivery	2
	Blood transfusion at any stage of labour	5
	Emergency general/spinal anaesthetic	5
	Intensive care not accounted for by any other factor	5
	Subtotal SECTION D	

TOTAL SCORES AND INDICATE CATEGORY AS SHOWN BELOW

Score 6	=	*Category I*	Score 14 - 18 =	*Category IV*
Score 7 - 9	=	*Category II*		
Score 10 - 13	=	*Category III*	Score 19+ =	*Category V*
			Other Categories	X A R

HAVE YOU CALCULATED LENGTH OF TIME IN DELIVERY SUITE ....?

* J A Ball Nuffield Institute *Leeds*

Section 3.2

Instructions on how to use the score system

1. Using the score system for women who have given birth

The scoring system has four sections:

A.   Gestation/labour/interventions

B.   Delivery

C.   Infant(s)

D.   Other intensive care factors.

At least six scores i.e. two each in sections A, B and C must be given to each mother/baby pair.

Scores are then given for any other indicator which is relevant to *either* mother or baby.

In all cases, once the scoring is complete:

- the scores are totalled *and*

- the category is ringed.

The length of time in the delivery suite is then calculated, rounded up to the nearest 15 minutes, and added to the bottom of the score sheet expressed in decimals e.g. 5 hours 5 minutes equals 5 hours, 5 hours 10 minutes is rounded up to 5 hours and 15 minutes (5.15).

2. Notes on completing the forms

LENGTH OF LABOUR
This includes time in labour *before* the woman came into the hospital, and is meant to reflect her degree of tiredness.

CONTINUOUS FETAL MONITORING
This does *not* mean initial or intermittent monitoring, but should be used for continuous electronic monitoring and/or sequential fetal blood sampling. It is meant to indicate concern about process of labour or suspected fetal distress.

CAESAREAN SECTIONS

These receive scores as follows:

- *Elective:* score 3 for elective anaesthetic in section A and 3 from section B.
- *Emergency:* score 5 from section B and 5 from section D for emergency anaesthetic.

Remember to score perineum for *all* caesarean sections (see also notes for hospitals without operating facilities on the delivery suite).

APGAR SCORES

This reflects any care required by the baby at delivery, therefore apgar score at five minutes should be used (see later note).

MULTIPLE BIRTHS

Scores should be given for each delivery, and each infant. If both babies are born by caesarean section, then one delivery is scored. If however, one is normal delivery and one is breech or caesarean section, then both deliveries are scored.

STILLBIRTHS (24 WEEKS GESTATION AND ABOVE)

Score apgar scores and birth weight e.g. Apgar less than 5 (score = 3), birth weight more than 2.5kg (score = 1), stillborn (score = 5) so total score for baby is nine.

DELIVERIES BEFORE 24 WEEKS OF GESTATION

If the infant is born alive, score all sections as for full term delivery. If the infant is not born alive, give scores for the mother only.

WOMEN WHOSE BABIES WERE BORN BEFORE ARRIVAL

Score all sections except for length of labour.

FLYING SQUADS, ESCORT DUTIES

Please see other information.

NOTE FOR APGAR SCORE

For units who do not use the Apgar System we suggest the following scores at five minutes after birth:

- Baby cries at birth, good colour   1
- Baby needs some assistance and is responding   2
- Baby gives rise to concern, poor colour, poor respiration, *etc*   3

3. Other categories and undelivered cases

For the following categories, there is no need to use the score system, simply indicate on the sheet whether or not the mother falls into category X, A or R. The length of time that the client has been in the delivery suite should be recorded as for delivered cases.

CATEGORY X

This category should be used for all mothers who are admitted to the delivery suite, but after assessment/monitoring are found not to be in labour or to need any intervention and are then sent home or transferred to another ward. For example, a woman comes in with some labour-like pain, but is not in labour, or a woman who comes in for monitoring, but does not require any further intervention.

Women who *do* require attention are included in Category A.

CATEGORY A

This category is used for women admitted as in Category X above but who require some intervention, including an intravenous infusion and/or monitoring prostin inductions e.g. antepartum haemorrhage, pre-eclampsia or premature labour.

If she then leaves the suite before delivery, she is classed as A. If however she eventually goes into labour and is delivered, then the normal score system should be used as she leaves the delivery suite.

CATEGORY R

This category is given to mothers who are re-admitted to the delivery suite for any reason, e.g. tubal ligation, examination under anaesthetic etc.

OTHER CASES/ACTIVITIES IN SOME DELIVERY SUITES

In some maternity units, flying squads, escorts may be a feature. Please see later information for gathering staff time for these situations.

Section 3.3

Recording time needed for midwifery care

Once the scores have been allocated and the category scored, the midwife should then add to the top of the score sheet the length of time the woman has been in the delivery suite or has received the attention of a midwife for established labour. Examples are given below.

1. *Direct admission to delivery suite*

   For example, the woman began her labour at home at 14.00 hours, and came into the delivery suite at 16.30 hours. She was then assessed and continued to labour until she delivered at 21.15 hours. Another hour and a half ensues whilst the midwife clears up, helps to put the baby on the breast, and deals with all the paperwork, transferring mother and baby to the postnatal ward at 22.45.

   Length of time in delivery suite/receiving midwifery care = 6.25 hours (16.30 - 22.45).

2. *Domino or caseload delivery where woman is first attended at home*

   A woman calls her midwife at 10.00 hours and the midwife attends at 10.15 hours. As labour is not yet established, she calls back again at 12.30 hours. The woman is now getting into established labour and her midwife transfers her to hospital at 13.45 hours. Delivery is at 20.00 hours, and another hour and a half ensues whilst the midwife clears up, helps to put the baby to the breast, and completes all the paperwork, etc, transferring mother and baby to the postnatal ward or to await transfer home at 21.30 hours.

   Length of time in delivery suite/receiving midwifery care = 9 hours (12.30 - 21.30).

3. *Antenatal wards*

   A woman may have been induced while on the antenatal ward, and later transferred to the delivery suite. Normally, this happens when labour is established but it may be that because of heavy workload on the delivery suite the woman is cared for in labour for some time on the antenatal ward.

   In this case, the length of time that the woman received care from a midwife should be calculated from the time that a partogram or other intrapartum record was commenced in the antenatal ward until the time of transfer back to a ward after delivery as before e.g. after overnight prostin a woman begins to have regular contractions on the ward at 11.00 hours, a partogram is commenced and she is regularly monitored before being transferred to the delivery suite at 13.10 hours. She delivers at 22.00 and is transferred to postnatal ward at 23.45 hours.

Her length of time in delivery suite/receiving midwifery care = 12.75 hours (11.00 - 23.45).

Remember to round up the minutes to quarters of an hour and express the length of time in decimals (especially if the data is going straight into a computer based record).

Hospitals without operating facilities on the delivery suite

EMERGENCY SECTION

When mothers have been in labour on the delivery suite and are then moved to an external theatre for caesarean section and escorted throughout by a midwife, who stays with the mother and baby until they are transferred to the postnatal ward, then the length of time spent equals all the time on delivery suite before transfer plus the time spent in the theatre.

ELECTIVE SECTION

If the mother is brought to the delivery suite for preparation, and then taken to theatre as above, then the time recorded should be the time from arriving on the suite to returning to the ward.

Flying squads/escorts

If a midwife/midwives go out with the flying squad or need to escort a mother in labour to another unit, then this should be separately recorded as follows.

On each occasion, note the time the midwife/midwives left the unit and the time they returned. The time out is then calculated. If more than one midwife is involved then the time is doubled e.g. flying squad called at 2.30am and returned at 5.15am = 2.75 hours. If two midwives were involved = 5.5 hours.

Section 3.4

Exercise for using the patient classification system in the delivery suite

You will find a number of case studies below.

Score each case using the system shown on the score sheet, classify the mother and baby, or babies, into the appropriate Birthrate category and then calculate the length of time in the delivery suite.

Then check your answers against those given at the end of the case studies.

---

1. Mrs Johnson

   Primigravida aged 32 years, admitted in labour at 07.30 hours.
   Gestation 41 weeks.

   Has had a healthy pregnancy and wishes to manage labour without drugs if possible. Fetal heart monitored electronically for one hour then discontinued.

   - Labour progressed well, mother coping well.

   - 14.00 hours. Second stage commenced. Fetal heart slowing and not picking up between contractions.

   - Episiotomy performed to speed delivery of head, normal delivery of little girl at 14.50 hours.

   - Apgar 8 at 5 minutes, birth weight 3.2 kgms.

   - Infant recovered well, crying lustily at 10 minutes old.

   - Put to breast, mother and dad delighted.

   - Mother's perineum sutured. Length of labour assessed at 9.25 hours.

   - Mother and baby transferred to postnatal ward at 16.35 hours.

---

2. Mrs Patel

Gravida 3 aged 24 years, has history of rheumatic heart fever and has been under the care of consultant physician during pregnancy. In order to reduce strain during second stage, elective forceps delivery has been recommended.

Mrs. Patel was admitted in labour at 09.50 hours. Gestation 36 weeks. She has grown up in England and there are no language problems. When admitted she has oedema of both feet and hands. Fetal heart monitored electronically throughout labour. In view of oedema the question of elective caesarean is raised, intravenous glucose is commenced and epidural given.

- Labour progressed well. Mother coping well, fetal condition is satisfactory.

- 13.20 hours: Second stage commenced. Elective forceps delivery performed with delivery of live boy at 13.40 hours.

- Episiotomy sutured, IVI maintained post-delivery.

- Baby: Apgar 8 at five minutes, birth weight 2.9 kgms.

- Put to breast, mother and dad delighted.

- Length of labour assessed at 7.25 hours.

- Mother and baby transferred to postnatal ward at 14.35 hours.

3. Mrs Parkes

Primigravida aged 17 years, admitted in labour at 12.20 hours. Gestation 39 weeks. She is accompanied by her mother, is rather scared and distressed by contractions. Pethidine given, does not want an epidural. Fetal heart remains satisfactory throughout labour.

- 15.00 hours, very distressed. Epidural given, IVI set up at same time. Contractions are not strong. At 18.00 Syntocinon added to IVI.

- 20.30 hours. Second stage commenced.

- 21.40 hours. Normal delivery of little girl.

- Apgar 8 at five minutes, birth weight 3.0 kgms. Perineum intact.

- Length of labour: 10.5 hours.

- Mother and baby transferred to postnatal ward at 22.55 hours.

4. Miss Roberts

Primigravida at 38 weeks gestation, admitted with backache and weak contractions at 20.30 hours.

On examination, contractions not felt, cervical os tightly closed but soft. Fetal heart satisfactory. Mother's BP 120/80.

Not considered to be in labour or in need of any treatment, sent to antenatal ward at 01.45 hours.

5. Mrs Marks

Gravida 2 aged 24 years, expecting twins, admitted in labour at 14.00 hours. Gestation 37 weeks.

- Presentation one vertex, one breech. Fetal hearts monitored electronically throughout labour.

- Labour progressed well, spontaneous rupture of membranes at 16.20 hours. Vaginal examination reveals prolapsed cord.

- Emergency caesarean section performed at 17.00 hours under general anaesthetic. Paediatrician present. Both babies born alive, both boys.

- Infant 1: Apgar 7 Birth weight 2.3 kgms

  Infant 2: Apgar 4, resuscitated, recovery fair, birth weight 2.5 kgms, transferred to SCBU.

- Length of labour: 6 hours; mother very sick after anaesthetic, IV set up during C/S, maintained post-delivery.

- Mother remained on delivery suite throughout the night.

- Transferred to postnatal ward at 09.15 hours on following day.

6. Mrs Jenkinson

Gravida 2, 40 weeks gestation, healthy pregnancy admitted at 15.20 hours in labour.

- Labour progressed well to second stage at 18.50 hours.

- Normal delivery of healthy boy at 19.15 hours, perineum intact.

- Baby: Apgar 8 at five minutes. Birth weight 3.25 kgms.

- Third stage: Placenta retained, mother's condition stable, blood loss minimal. I.V. infusion set up.

- Manual removal under general anaesthetic at 19.50 hours.

- Length of labour assessed as 7 hours. Recovery satisfactory, mother and baby transferred to postnatal ward at 21.00 hours.

Answers to case studies:

	A	**B**	**C**	**D**	**TOTAL**	**CATEGORY**	**TIME (hours)**
Johnson	3	3	2	-	8	II	9
Patel	16	4	2	-	22	V	4.75
Parkes	8	2	2	-	12	III	10.75
Roberts	CATEGORY X					X	
Marks	9	6	8	5	28	V	19.5
Jenkinson	2	2	2	7	13	III	5.75

The scores show how all the different events are allowed for and if you analyse the scores in each section you can make some judgements about the quality/effectiveness of the intrapartum care received e.g. Mrs Patel who was in intensive care during labour led to a good outcome or how with Mrs Jenkinson an unexpected crisis can follow a normal labour and delivery.

Section 3.5

Setting up the system and ensuring reliability of data

Setting the system up

All midwives should be made aware of the principles and use of the system. Make sure that all part-time and agency or bank staff are included. Reliability checks should be carried out to ensure that the system is not being misused (see later notes).

Collating the daily and monthly data

THE DAILY DATA

(i)   The midwife responsible for the care of each client should complete a score sheet before transferring her client to the ward. The scores are checked, the category is indicated and the length of time the woman spent in the delivery suite is recorded.

(ii)   The completed sheet is then put in the current day's folder, and the length of stay is recorded on a sheet for the category to which the mother has been assigned by her scores (e.g. all the Category I, II etc.).

(iii)   A time for daily census of workload is agreed e.g. 18.00 hours or 22.00 hours, and the same time is used each day.

At the agreed time, the following action is taken:

1.   Collect all the forms and sort them into each Category I-V, X, A and R.
2.   Enter the number of cases per category for that day upon the monthly record sheet (see example opposite) or into computer spreadsheet.
3.   Check that a time report has been recorded on the appropriate category sheet for each client in each category.
4.   Any mothers who are still in the delivery suite at the time agreed for the daily workload census to be taken should be entered upon the next day's workload census.

COLLATING THE MONTHLY DATA

At the end of each month, the following data is produced:
(i)   the number and case mix of clients
(ii)   the mean time in the delivery suite per category.

(i)   Number and case mix:

- total the number of cases in each category
- calculate the percentage of cases per category
- calculate the *daily mean number* of cases per category.

For example, in June there were 178 delivered cases. The number and percentages for each category were:

Category I	Category II	Category III	Category IV	Category V	TOTAL
31	75	29	17	26	178
17.4%	42.1%	16.3%	9.6%	14.6%	100%

For other cases, the numbers and percentages were:

Category X	Category A	Category R	TOTAL
36	10	2	48
75%	20.8%	4.2%	100%

The daily mean average number of cases per category over 30 days was:

- Category I   1.0 cases
- Category II   2.5 cases
- Category III   1.0 cases
- Category IV   0.6 cases
- Category V   0.9 cases
- Category X   1.2 cases
- Category A   0.3 cases
- Category R   0.1 cases

The daily mean number of cases per category will form the major part of the workload calculations.

(ii)   Mean time per category:
•   Note the lowest and the highest time recorded (range)
•   Calculate the mean time per category by dividing the total hours recorded by the number of cases recorded.

In June, 75 Category II cases are recorded. The shortest length of time is 4.5 hours, the longest is 18.5 hours (range).

For example, the total time for 75 cases is 526 hours/75 cases so the mean time per Category III case equals seven hours.

The mean time per category recorded will provide the time element in the workforce calculation.

Remember to use the correct number of days per month (28 - 31).

(iii)   Flying squads
When these are recorded, produce mean number per month and average time per case/situation in the same way.

Ensuring reliability

This can be checked by randomly selecting ten per cent of all *Birthrate* score sheets per category each month, and comparing the scores given, the calculation of category and the time in the delivery suite against the case record.

If any discrepancies are found, they should be brought to the attention of the midwife who completed the score sheet. If persistent faults are found, this indicates misunderstanding of the system and all staff should be informed of the problem arising and necessary corrections made.

Section 3.6

Using the data
1. Turning data into midwives (workforce planning)
2. Cautions and other issues
3. Reviewing outcomes

Workforce planning
1. Calculating the staff required to meet the workload for delivered cases

The data collected in each unit will reflect that unit's usual patterns of work i.e. the volume and case-mix it currently deals with.

Most of the data shown below are drawn from *real* hospitals who have implemented *Birthrate*.

a)   Number and case-mix of delivered cases:
      At the end of a minimum of six months collection of verified data, the mean number of cases per category and the percentages per category should be calculated as discussed earlier.

A typical example is shown in Table 3.1 below (one year's data):

Table 3.1	BIRTHRATE CATEGORIES					
	I	II	III	IV	V	VI
% Case mix	10.8	36.9	19.2	14.2	18.9	100
No. cases per annum	324	1107	576	426	567	3000
Daily means no. cases	0.89	3.03	1.58	1.17	1.55	8.22

b)   How many midwife hours per category?
The monthly data sheets produce the mean time spent by the client in the delivery suite. This forms the basis of the mean time required per category, together with percentage increases of midwife time required for the care of more complicated cases III, IV and V.

The mean midwife time for these cases is increased by 20 per cent, 30 per cent and 40 per cent respectively. This can easily be accomplished by multiplying the mean hours by 1.2, 1.3 or 1.4.

The results are shown in Table 3.2 below.

Table 3.2	**CALCULATING MIDWIFE TIME NEEDED PER CATEGORY**			
	Mean hours per category	% Midwife time needed	Total hours	Workload ratios per category
I	4.9	100%	4.9	1.0 baseline
II	7.35	100%	7.35	1.5
III	9.42	120%	11.3	2.3
IV	12.42	130%	16.15	3.3
V	17.15	140%	24.01	4.9

Caution: Table 3.2 shows midwife hours less than 4.9 for Category I
Experience has shown that where all intrapartum care has been captured and there is no policy of augmenting or inducing all labours (see later discussion on quality issues) then one would expect a mean time per Category I to be around or slightly above five hours per case. If it is much less than this, then make sure that all care is being captured e.g. time spent in labour and midwife in attendance at home or on an antenatal ward.

Workload ratios and indices

Table 3.2 shows workload ratios in the last column. Using such ratios make it easier to use a staffing formula because it reduces the number of calculations (see below). The workload index is also useful as a sensitive indicator of change in workload month by month, or when some significant change in clinical policies occurs.

To work these out always take Category I as the baseline.

Therefore, as you can see in Table 3.2, 7.35 hours/4.9 = 1.5.

The workload index indicates changes in either the volume or the case mix of clients being cared for. The following details are given.

The data shown in Tables 3.1 and 3.2 are now used to calculate the staff required (midwives only):

Table 3.3	**BIRTHRATE CATEGORIES**					
	I	II	III	IV	V	Total
% Case mix	10.8	36.9	19.2	14.2	18.9	100
No. cases per annum	324	1107	576	426	567	3000
Daily mean no. cases	0.89	3.03	1.58	1.17	1.55	8.22
Workload ratios	1.0	1.5	2.3	3.3	4.9	
Workload index	0.89	4.55	3.63	3.86	7.6	20.53

The *workload index* is gained by multiplying the daily mean number of cases per category with the workload ratios which arise from the midwife time required per category.

The *total workload index* represents the total workload produced from the number and case-mix shown. It really means that the total workload is equal to 20.53 Category I cases per day.

Calculating staff

1. Delivered cases

If workload index is 20.53 Category I cases per day and each Category I case needs 4.9 hours of midwife time, then the daily midwife hours needed are:

- 20.53 x 4.9 = 100.6 midwife hours per day
- 100.6 x 7 = 704 midwife hours needed per week.

These hours represent the time needed for all direct and indirect care of clients, including paper work.

To this should be added further allowances:

1.   Add 15 per cent variance to allow for unpredictability of workload, plus some staff personal time and tuition of students over and above that given during the care of clients **(704 x 1.15 = 809.81 midwife hours per week).**

2.   A further five per cent is added to delivered cases workload only to allow for ward/unit administration, staff meetings, etc **(809.81 x 1.05 = 850.30 midwife hours per week).**

     We now have the total midwife hours per week day and night which is required to care for the workload shown in Table 3. This is divided by 37.5 to produce the in-post staffing figure **(850.30/37.5 = 22.67 w.t.e. midwives).**

3.   A further allowance of 17.3 per cent should now be added to allow for holidays, and a small amount of sickness/study leave to produce the total establishment staffing figures **(22.67 w.t.e x 1.173 = 26.59 w.t.e.).**

How much for holidays and sick leave

In the example given above, 17.3 per cent has been added for holidays. This is based on five weeks annual leave plus ten days bank holiday which amounts to seven weeks.

Add two further weeks for sickness and small amount of study leave which equals a minimum of nine weeks per annum when a midwife is off-duty.

*   9 weeks = 17.3 per cent of 52 weeks (9/52 x 100 = 17.3 per cent).

It may be that in your working situation different allowances are given, in which case provided *it is not less than that given above, you should use your own percentage allowance to calculate holidays, sickness and study leave allowances.*

Maternity leave

It is not possible, or feasible, to add any percentage allowances for maternity leave to the total staffing formula. Maternity leave is extremely variable from year to year and does not affect all staff. Therefore, managers are advised to calculate staff as needed and to make their own adjustment for maternity leave where this can be accurately predicted in any given timescale.

Further staff may be needed for care of other categories X, A R and flying squad, escort, off-site theatre duties, etc., where applicable.

2. What is the data telling you

It is possible to identify the impact of changes in clinical practice where these occur, and this should be taken into consideration when assessing staffing needs.

Table 3.4	BIRTHRATE CATEGORIES: Monthly figures					
	I	II	III	IV	V	Total
January	33	78	34	30	40	215
February	25	61	44	36	36	202
March	25	66	55	40	37	
April	31	52	68	38	41	230
May	27	47	72	38	45	229
June	31	45	74	42	35	227
TOTALS	172	349	347	224	234	1326

These figures show a very consistent number of deliveries per month but there is a move to Category III from Categories I and II which came about when the epidural service was extended in April.

The same midwife time per category was applied for each month as shown in Tables 3.2 and 3.3 previously, but because of the change in the case mix, the workload indices for each month were as follows:

Month	No. days	Workload index	In post w.t.e.	TOTAL w.t.e.
January	31	16.88	18.52	21.73
February	28	18.32	20.11	23.58
March	31	18.19	19.96	23.42
April	30	19.72	21.65	25.39
May	31	19.65	21.56	25.29
June	30	19.25	21.18	24.84

Normally, staffing calculations would be based on six months data which in the case of Table 3.4 would result in:

- Workload index: 18.67 (mean index produced for indices for each month)
- In post: 20.49 w.t.e.
- Total est.: 24.04 w.t.e.

However, the manager would be wise to assess her needs on the basis of the latter three months and then to review in three months time when a full six months data under the new care policy is available e.g. on April - June figures:

- Workload index: 19.54 (mean index on April-June only)
- In post: 21.46 w.t.e.
- Total est. 25.17 w.t.e.

3. Calculating the staff needed for other cases/workload

X, A, R AND FLYING SQUAD

It has been found that it is easier to calculate staff needed by using total/mean hours per case only. Workload ratios are no longer used in view of the comparatively small numbers involved.

For *Categories A and R, escort* or *flying squad* the total time is used.

However, in the case of Category X cases, experience has shown that they do not need the total attention of a midwife, and the time spent on the delivery suite varied from half an hour to 15 or more hours.

In terms of efficient use of midwife time therefore, it is recommended that an allowance of one hour per Category X case is allocated. This would assume that Category X clients need a midwife for half of the time spent in the delivery (actual time is two hours) and would then be either transferred to a ward or home.

The calculations needed for Category A are as follows:

No. cases over six months	48
Mean hours per case	15.2
TOTAL HOURS	729.6
Weekly hours *	28.06
+ 15% variance	32.37
In post **	0.86 w.t.e
+17.3% **TOTAL ESTABLISHMENT**	1.01 w.t.e.
** 5 per cent administration allowance **is not** added to other cases	
* divide total by 26 weeks, or in the case of annual figures by 52 weeks	

For Category R:

No. cases over six months	35
Mean hours per case	2.6
TOTAL HOURS	91.0
Weekly hours *	3.5
+ 15 % variance	4.03
In post **	0.11 w.t.e
+17.3% **TOTAL ESTABLISHMENT**	0.13 w.t.e.
* divide by 26 weeks, or in the case of annual figures by 52 weeks	
** 5 per cent administration allowance **is not** added to other cases	

For Category X:

No. cases over six months	386
Mean hours per case	1.0
TOTAL HOURS	386
Weekly hours*	14.85
+ 15% variance	17.07
In post**	0.46 w.t.e.
+17.3% **TOTAL ESTABLISHMENT**	0.53 w.t.e.
* divide total by 26 weeks, or in the case of annual figures by 52 weeks	
** 5 per cent administration allowance **is not** added to other cases	

Flying squad etc. are calculated in the same way:

No. cases over six months	5
Mean hours per case	4.6
TOTAL HOURS	23.0
Weekly hours	0.88
+ 15 % variance	1.01
In post	0.03 w.t.e
+ 17.3% **TOTAL ESTABLISHMENT**	0.03 w.t.e.

TOTAL STAFF FOR OTHER CASES	
In post 1.46 w.t.e	Total establishment 1.71 w.t.e.

Total staff needed on case-mix shown in Table 3.1 plus allowances for extra cases.

INTRAPARTUM CARE
- **In post 22.67** w.t.e plus extra cases X, A, R and flying squad = **1.46 w.t.e.** = total of **24.13 w.t.e.**
- When 17.3 per cent is added = total establishment of **28.3 w.t.e.**

These figures are for midwives only!

Caution:
In some cases the total establishment will be smaller than the numbers needed to run a delivery suite on two or three shifts around the 24 hours. Managers who find this result should not panic or reject *Birthrate*. This is the situation where staff in excess of workload assessed needs are justified to provide a 24 hour service and this will be discussed later. This need is acknowledged in other work, notably that of the Audit Commission report on nursing workload systems (Ball et al, 1989; Audit Commission, 1992).

Section 3.7

Examples and exercises in calculating staff

In the next section we have two separate exercises which illustrate the use of *Birthrate* data, and the difference that case-mix and volume of workload can make on the number of staff needed.

The first set show how different care policies make a notable difference to the numbers of midwives needed, even though the total number of cases per month are the same.

The next two exercises give you real data from two different sized hospitals.

What we want you to do

Work out the staffing requirements based on the data provided and using the formula given (which was given earlier in this section). Then check your results against the answers given at the end of this section.

Exercise One: same number, different case-mix

Following you will find the workload data for four fictitious units who all have 100 cases per month, but you have different care policies and thus different case-mixes.

(i) **Washbrook Hospital** has *no* epidural service after 8.00pm or at weekends/ bank holidays

Midwives needed for intrapartum care

CASEMIX CLASSIFIED INTO BIRTHRATE OUTCOME CATEGORIES						
	I	II	III	IV	V	TOTAL
% Case Mix	25.8	25.6	13.5	15.8	19.3	100
Annual Number	*825.60*	*819.20*	*432.00*	*505.60*	*617.60*	*3200*
Daily Mean	2.26	2.24	1.18	1.39	1.69	8.77
Workload Ratio	*1.00*	*1.40*	*2.40*	*3.20*	*4.80*	
Workload Index	2.26	3.14	2.84	4.45	8.11	20.80

Allowing 5.2 midwife hours per Category I work out the staffing requirements based on this case mix:

- Midwife hours per day

- Midwife hours per week

- *Add 15 per cent allowance for variability*

- *Add 5 per cent for management: audit, meetings, etc*

- IN POST W.T.E. STAFF NEEDED =

- *Add 17.3 per cent holidays/sickness/study leave*

FULL ESTABLISHMENT: W.T.E. STAFF NEEDED =

(ii)   **Rosaleen Steele Hospital** has a 24 hour epidural service.

Midwives needed for intrapartum care

CASEMIX CLASSIFIED INTO BIRTHRATE OUTCOME CATEGORIES						
	I	II	III	IV	V	TOTAL
% Case Mix	15.8	25.6	22.4	16.9	19.3	100
Annual Number	*505.60*	*819.20*	*716.80*	*540.80*	*617.60*	*3200*
Daily Mean	1.39	2.24	1.96	1.48	1.69	8.77
Workload Ratio	*1.00*	*1.40*	*2.40*	*3.20*	*4.80*	
Workload Index	1.39	3.14	4.70	4.74	8.11	22.10

Allowing 5.2 midwife hours per Category I work out the staffing requirements based on this case mix:

- Midwife hours per day

- Midwife hours per week

- *Add 15 per cent allowance for variability*

- *Add 5 per cent for management: audit, meetings, etc*

- IN POST W.T.E. STAFF NEEDED =

- *Add 17.3 per cent holidays/sickness/study leave*

FULL ESTABLISHMENT: W.T.E. STAFF NEEDED =

(iii)　**Jean Ball Unit** still has a very active management style, with a high induction and caesarean section rate and a 24 hour epidural service.

Midwives needed for intrapartum care

CASEMIX CLASSIFIED INTO BIRTHRATE OUTCOME CATEGORIES						
	I	II	III	IV	V	TOTAL
% Case Mix	13.7	17.4	23.5	18.1	27.3	100
Annual Number	*438.40*	*556.80*	*752.00*	*579.20*	*873.60*	*3200*
Daily Mean	1.20	1.53	2.06	1.59	2.39	8.77
Workload Ratio	*1.00*	*1.40*	*2.40*	*3.20*	*4.80*	
Workload Index	1.20	2.14	4.94	5.08	11.47	24.83

Allowing 5.2 midwife hours per Category I work out the staffing requirements based on this case mix:

- Midwife hours per day

- Midwife hours per week

- *Add 15 per cent allowance for variability*

- *Add 5 per cent for management: audit, meetings, etc*

- IN POST W.T.E. STAFF NEEDED =

- *Add 17.3 per cent holidays/sickness/study leave*

FULL ESTABLISHMENT: W.T.E. STAFF NEEDED =

(iv)   **Nicholas Winterton Unit** is mainly midwife managed, with a birth pool and 24 hour epidural service. Consultants care for high risk cases, moderate caesarean rate.

Midwives needed for intrapartum care

CASEMIX CLASSIFIED INTO BIRTHRATE OUTCOME CATEGORIES						
	I	II	III	IV	V	TOTAL
% Case Mix	18.4	22.6	22.4	17	19.6	100
Annual Number	*588.80*	*723.20*	*716.80*	*544.00*	*627.20*	*3200*
Daily Mean	1.61	1.98	1.96	1.49	1.72	8.77
Workload Ratio	*1.00*	*1.40*	*2.40*	*3.20*	*4.80*	
Workload Index	1.61	2.77	4.71	4.77	8.25	22.12

Allowing 5.2 midwife hours per Category I work out the staffing requirements based on this case mix:

- Midwife hours per day

- Midwife hours per week

- *Add 15 per cent allowance for variability*

- *Add 5 per cent for management: audit, meetings, etc*

- IN POST W.T.E. STAFF NEEDED =

- *Add 17.3 per cent holidays/sickness/study leave*

- FULL ESTABLISHMENT: W.T.E. STAFF NEEDED =

Exercise Two

Cathedral City and Parkham Hospitals contain real data gained in 1992 and 1994.

Work out the staffing numbers based on the data given, and this time add in that required for X, A, R and escort duties.

Cathedral City Hospital 1992: Exercise in calculating staff

Midwives needed for intrapartum care

CASEMIX CLASSIFIED INTO BIRTHRATE OUTCOME CATEGORIES						
	I	II	III	IV	V	TOTAL
% Case Mix	10.80	36.90	19.20	14.20	18.90	100
Annual Number	*324.00*	*1107.00*	*576.00*	*426.00*	*567.00*	*3000*
Daily Mean	0.89	3.03	1.58	1.17	1.55	8.22
Workload Ratio	*1.00*	*1.34*	*2.14*	*2.60*	*4.20*	
Workload Index	0.89	4.06	3.38	3.04	6.51	17.88

TOTAL WORKLOAD INDEX   17.88

- Mean hours per Category I | 5.90 |

- Midwife hours per day

- Midwife hours per week

- *Add 15 per cent allowance for variability*

- *Add 5 per cent for management: audit, meetings, etc*

- IN POST W.T.E. STAFF NEEDED   =

- *Add 17.3 per cent holidays/sickness/study leave*

FULL ESTABLISHMENT: W.T.E. STAFF NEEDED =

Cathedral City Hospital: Data on X, A, R and escorts per annum

Midwives needed for other categories

CATEGORY X	
No. per annum	736.00
Mid. hrs per case	1.00
Annual hours	736.00
Mid. hrs per week	
+15 % variance	
In post w.t.e.	
+ 17.3% hols, etc	
TOTAL est. w.t.e/	

CATEGORY A	
No. per annum	53.00
Mid. hrs per case	18.30
Annual hours	
Mid. hrs per week	
+15% variance	
In post w.t.e.	
+ 17.3% hols, etc	
TOTAL est. w.t.e/	

CATEGORY R	
No. per annum	35.00
Mid. hrs per case	9.00
Annual hours	
Mid. hrs per week	
+15% variance	
In post w.t.e.	
+ 17.3% hols, etc	
TOTAL est. w.t.e/	

ESCORTS	
No. per annum	13.00
Mid. hrs per case	4.20
Annual hours	
Mid. hrs per week	
+15% variance	
In post w.t.e.	
+ 17.3% hols, etc	
TOTAL est. w.t.e/	

TOTAL STAFF REQUIRED FOR OTHER CASES:

In post [   ]   *Total establishment* [   ]

Parkham County Hospital 1992: Exercise in calculating staff

Midwives needed for intrapartum care

CASEMIX CLASSIFIED INTO BIRTHRATE OUTCOME CATEGORIES						
	I	II	III	IV	V	TOTAL
% Case Mix	7.8	23.2	32.5	18.7	17.8	100
Annual Number	*109.0*	*325.0*	*455.0*	*262.0*	*249.0*	*1400*
Daily Mean	0.3	0.9	1.2	0.7	0.7	3.8
Workload Ratio	*1.0*	*1.4*	*2.4*	*3.2*	*4.8*	
Workload Index	0.3	1.26	2.88	2.24	3.36	10.04

TOTAL WORKLOAD INDEX 10.04

- Mean hours per Category I | 4.30 |

- Midwife hours per day

- Midwife hours per week

- *Add 15 per cent allowance for variability*

- *Add 5 per cent for management: audit, meetings, etc*

- IN POST W.T.E. STAFF NEEDED =

- *Add 17.3 per cent holidays/sickness/study leave*

FULL ESTABLISHMENT: W.T.E STAFF NEEDED =

Parkham County Hospital: Data on X, A, R and escorts per annum

Midwives needed for other categories

CATEGORY X	
No. per annum	547.00
Mid. hrs per case	1.00
Annual hours	547.00
Mid. hrs per week	
+15% variance	
In post w.t.e.	
+ 17.3% hols, etc	
TOTAL est. w.t.e/	

CATEGORY A	
No. per annum	109.00
Mid. hrs per case	15.4
Annual hours	
Mid. hrs per week	
+15% variance	
In post w.t.e.	
+ 17.3% hols, etc	
TOTAL est. w.t.e/	

CATEGORY R	
No. per annum	15.00
Mid. hrs per case	7.5
Annual hours	
Mid. hrs per week	
+15% variance	
In post w.t.e.	
+ 17.3% hols, etc	
TOTAL est. w.t.e/	

ESCORTS	
No. per annum	10.00
Mid. hrs per case	5.00
Annual hours	
Mid. hrs per week	
+15% variance	
In post w.t.e.	
+ 17.3% hols, etc	
TOTAL est. w.t.e/	

TOTAL STAFF REQUIRED FOR OTHER CASES:

In post ☐   *Total establishment* ☐

What are the answers?

If your answers vary by a small margin, say a decimal point, then don't worry.

If however they vary quite a bit from those given below, then you need to re-check your arithmetic.

Details of the worked out results are shown at the end of this section.

Exercise One: same numbers, different case-mix

The answers may surprise you. Although each of the units had 100 deliveries for the month, they need different numbers of staff because of the differences in care patterns:

- Washbrook Unit needs 28.6 w.t.e. midwives (but is short of a full epidural service).

- Rosaleen Steele Unit provides a 24 hour epidural service so more women are able to make this choice and the unit therefore needs 30.38 w.t.e. midwives.

- Jean Ball Unit needs 34.14 w.t.e. midwives (because of very active management style).

- Nicholas Winterton Unit needs 30.41 w.t.e. midwives.

Exercise Two

Cathedral City needs 27.9 w.t.e. for delivered cases and 1.44 w.t.e. for X, A, R and escort duties. In fact escort duties are very minor, requiring only 0.04 w.t.e., but it is wise to record this work simply to demonstrate that although it is disruptive when it occurs, it does not require large numbers of staff to accommodate it.

Parkham County needs 11.41 w.t.e. for delivered cases and 1.65 w.t.e for X, A, R and escort duties. This is a good example of the other issues facing small maternity units. 11.41 w.t.e. would only just provide two midwives per shift with no lee-way for peaks of workload or troughs of staff sickness. How to manage this situation will be discussed in the next section.

Now check your results with the worked out answers…

Answers to Exercise One

(i)   **Washbrook Hospital** has *no* epidural service after 8.00pm or at weekends/ bank holidays

Midwives needed for intrapartum care

CASEMIX CLASSIFIED INTO BIRTHRATE OUTCOME CATEGORIES						
	I	II	III	IV	V	TOTAL
% Case Mix	25.8	25.6	13.5	15.8	19.3	100
Annual Number	*825.60*	*819.20*	*432.00*	*505.60*	*617.60*	*3200*
Daily Mean	2.26	2.24	1.18	1.39	1.69	8.77
Workload Ratio	*1.00*	*1.40*	*2.40*	*3.20*	*4.80*	
Workload Index	2.26	3.14	2.84	4.45	8.11	20.80

Allowing 5.2 midwife hours per Category I… *work out the staffing requirements based on this case mix:*

•	Midwife hours per day	108.16
•	Midwife hours per week	757.12
•	*Add 15 per cent allowance for variability*	870.69
•	*Add 5 per cent for management: audit, meetings, etc*	914.22
•	IN POST W.T.E. STAFF NEEDED =	24.38
•	*Add 17.3 per cent holidays/sickness/study leave*	28.60
FULL ESTABLISHMENT: W.T.E. STAFF NEEDED =		**28.60**

(ii)   **Rosaleen Steele Hospital** has a 24 hour epidural service

Midwives needed for intrapartum care

CASEMIX CLASSIFIED INTO BIRTHRATE OUTCOME CATEGORIES						
	I	II	III	IV	V	TOTAL
% Case Mix	15.8	25.6	22.4	16.9	19.3	100
Annual Number	*505.60*	*819.20*	*716.80*	*540.80*	*617.60*	*3200*
Daily Mean	1.39	2.24	1.96	1.48	1.69	8.77
Workload Ratio	*1.00*	*1.40*	*2.40*	*3.20*	*4.80*	
Workload Index	1.39	3.14	4.70	4.74	8.11	22.10

Allowing 5.2 midwife hours per Category I... *work out the staffing requirements based on this case mix:*

• Midwife hours per day	114.92
• Midwife hours per week	804.44
• *Add 15 per cent allowance for variability*	925.11
• *Add 5 per cent for management: audit, meetings, etc*	971.36
• IN POST W.T.E. STAFF NEEDED =	25.90
• Add 17.3 per cent holidays/sickness/study leave	30.38
FULL ESTABLISHMENT: W.T.E. STAFF NEEDED =	**30.38**

(iii) **Jean Ball Unit** still has a very active management style, with a high induction and caesarean section rate: 24 hour epidural service

Midwives needed for intrapartum care

CASEMIX CLASSIFIED INTO BIRTHRATE OUTCOME CATEGORIES						
	I	II	III	IV	V	TOTAL
% Case Mix	13.7	17.4	23.5	18.1	27.3	100
Annual Number	*438.40*	*556.80*	*752.00*	*579.20*	*873.60*	*3200*
Daily Mean	1.20	1.53	2.06	1.59	2.39	8.77
Workload Ratio	*1.00*	*1.40*	*2.40*	*3.20*	*4.80*	
Workload Index	1.20	2.14	4.94	5.08	11.47	24.83

Allowing 5.2 midwife hours per Category I... *work out the staffing requirements based on this case mix:*

• Midwife hours per day	129.12
• Midwife hours per week	903.81
• *Add 15 per cent allowance for variability*	1039.86
• *Add 5 per cent for management: audit, meetings, etc*	1091.35
• IN POST W.T.E. STAFF NEEDED =	29.10
• *Add 17.3 per cent holidays/sickness/study leave*	34.14
FULL ESTABLISHMENT: W.T.E. STAFF NEEDED =	**34.14**

(iv) **Nicholas Winterton Unit** is mainly midwife managed, with birth pool, etc. 24 hours epidural service. Consultants care for high risk cases, moderate caesarean rate.

Midwives needed for intrapartum care

CASEMIX CLASSIFIED INTO BIRTHRATE OUTCOME CATEGORIES						
	I	II	III	IV	V	TOTAL
% Case Mix	18.4	22.6	22.4	17	19.6	100
Annual Number	*588.80*	*723.20*	*716.80*	*544.00*	*627.20*	*3200*
Daily Mean	1.61	1.98	1.96	1.49	1.72	8.77
Workload Ratio	*1.00*	*1.40*	*2.40*	*3.20*	*4.80*	
Workload Index	1.61	2.77	4.70	4.77	8.25	22.12

Allowing 5.2 midwife hours per Category I... *work out the staffing requirements based on this case mix:*

• Midwife hours per day	115.02
• Midwife hours per week	805.14
• *Add 15 per cent allowance for variability*	925.91
• *Add 5 per cent for management: audit, meetings, etc*	972.21
• IN POST W.T.E. STAFF NEEDED =	25.93
• Add 17.3 per cent holidays/sickness/study leave	30.41
FULL ESTABLISHMENT: W.T.E. STAFF NEEDED =	**30.41**

Exercise Two

Cathedral City Hospital: Exercise in calculating staff

Midwives needed for intrapartum care

CASEMIX CLASSIFIED INTO BIRTHRATE OUTCOME CATEGORIES						
	I	II	III	IV	V	TOTAL
% Case Mix	10.80	36.90	19.20	14.20	18.90	100
Annual Number	*324.00*	*1107.00*	*576.00*	*426.00*	*567.00*	*3000*
Daily Mean	0.89	3.03	1.58	1.17	1.55	8.22
Workload Ratio	*1.00*	*1.34*	*2.14*	*2.60*	*4.20*	
Workload Index	0.89	4.06	3.38	3.04	6.51	17.88

TOTAL WORKLOAD INDEX	17.88

- Mean hours per Category I — 5.90
- Midwife hours per day — 105.49
- Midwife hours per week — 738.43
- *Add 15 per cent allowance for variability* — 849.19
- *Add 5 per cent for management: audit, meetings, etc* — 891.65
- IN POST W.T.E. STAFF NEEDED = — 23.78
- *Add 17.3 per cent holidays/sickness/study leave* — 27.90

FULL ESTABLISHMENT: W.T.E. STAFF NEEDED = — **27.90**

Data on X, A, R and escorts per annum

Midwives needed for other categories:

CATEGORY X	
No per annum	736.00
Mid. hrs per case	1.00
Annual hours	736.00
Mid. hrs per week	14.15
+15% variance	16.28
In post w.t.e.	0.43
+ 17.3% hols, etc	0.51
TOTAL est. w.t.e/	0.51

CATEGORY A	
No per annum	53.00
Mid. hrs per case	18.30
Annual hours	969.90
Mid. hrs per week	18.65
+15% variance	21.45
In post w.t.e.	0.57
+ 17.3% hols, etc	0.67
TOTAL est. w.t.e/	0.67

CATEGORY R	
No per annum	35.00
Mid. hrs per case	9.00
Annual hours	315.00
Mid. hrs per week	6.06
+15% variance	6.97
In post w.t.e.	0.19
+ 17.3% hols, etc	0.22
TOTAL est. w.t.e/	0.22

ESCORTS	
No per annum	13.00
Mid. hrs per case	4.20
Annual hours	54.60
Mid. hrs per week	1.05
+15% variance	1.21
In post w.t.e.	0.03
+ 17.3% hols, etc	0.04
TOTAL est. w.t.e/	0.04

TOTAL STAFF REQUIRED FOR OTHER CASES:

In post 1.22   *Total establishment* 1.44

Parkham County Hospital 1992: exercise in calculating staff

Midwives needed for intrapartum care

CASEMIX CLASSIFIED INTO BIRTHRATE OUTCOME CATEGORIES						
	I	II	III	IV	V	TOTAL
% Case Mix	7.8	23.2	32.5	18.7	17.8	100
Annual Number	*109.0*	*325.0*	*455.0*	*262.0*	*249.0*	*1400*
Daily Mean	0.3	0.9	1.2	0.7	0.7	3.8
Workload Ratio	*1.0*	*1.4*	*2.4*	*3.2*	*4.8*	
Workload Index	0.3	1.26	2.88	2.24	3.36	10.04

TOTAL WORKLOAD INDEX   10.04

•	Mean hours per Category I	4.30
•	Midwife hours per day	43.17
•	Midwife hours per week	302.20
•	*Add 15 per cent allowance for variability*	347.53
•	*Add 5 per cent for management: audit, meetings, etc*	364.91
•	IN POST W.T.E. STAFF NEEDED =	9.73
•	*Add 17.3 per cent holidays/sickness/study leave*	11.41
	FULL ESTABLISHMENT: W.T.E. STAFF NEEDED =	**11.41**

Data on X, A, R and escorts per annum

Midwives needed for other categories:

CATEGORY X	
No per annum	547.00
Mid. hrs per case	1.00
Annual hours	547.00
Mid. hrs per week	10.52
+15% variance	12.10
In post w.t.e.	0.32
+ 17.3% hols, etc	0.38
TOTAL est. w.t.e/	0.38

CATEGORY A	
No per annum	109.00
Mid. hrs per case	15.40
Annual hours	1678.60
Mid. hrs per week	32.38
+15% variance	37.12
In post w.t.e.	0.99
+ 17.3% hols, etc	1.16
TOTAL est. w.t.e/	1.16

CATEGORY R	
No per annum	15.00
Mid. hrs per case	7.5
Annual hours	112.5
Mid. hrs per week	2.16
+15% variance	2.48
In post w.t.e.	0.07
+ 17.3% hols, etc	0.08
TOTAL est. w.t.e/	0.08

ESCORTS	
No per annum	10.00
Mid. hrs per case	5.00
Annual hours	50.00
Mid. hrs per week	0.96
+15% variance	1.11
In post w.t.e.	0.03
+ 17.3% hols, etc	0.035
TOTAL est. w.t.e/	0.035

TOTAL STAFF REQUIRED FOR OTHER CASES :

In post 1.40   *Total establishment* 1.65

Section 3.8

Making management judgements on the results

In the introduction we outlined the processes required for sound service and workforce planning.

In Section 1, assessing the demand has shown the need to assess the *Birthrate* data results by appraisal of quality issues, and any other variations needed. We can see this process beginning in the exercises we have just completed.

Exercise One

If you were the midwifery manager of Washbrook Unit you could put a good case forward for an increase in staff to enable a 24 hour epidural service to begin, and if you managed Jean Ball Unit you might want to persuade the consultants to adopt a less interventionist approach by suggesting that this would enable a reduction in staff as well as benefitting the mothers. Similarly, the manager of Nicholas Winterton could demonstrate that midwifery managed care was not costing more than conventional care patterns.

This illustrates, albeit tentatively, the way in which *Birthrate* data can inform quality issues.

Exercise Two

Parkham Unit manager must now work out how many staff are needed per shift to provide a satisfactory standard of midwife cover, but she might be able to increase the workload to make good use of this increased staffing, by taking clients who need some day time antenatal care monitoring, Category X, etc. If the need to deploy more staff than indicated by workload is found in the rest of the unit, then the manager needs to recognize that she has spare capacity available and should seek to attract new clients from other areas.

Reviewing care policies for Category X clients

In almost all the units which have implemented *Birthrate*, it has been found that Category X clients form a large percentage of all admissions to delivery suites, and this raises a number of issues.

The following list shows the percentages found in the trial of the system in seven hospitals in Trent Region in 1986/87 (three months data).

	Category X Number	% of all admissions
Unit A	365	23.4
Unit B	349	29.1
Unit C	728	32.0
Unit D	280	28.8
Unit E	484	36.7
Unit F	508	27.3
Unit G	543	29.9 (Ball, 1992)

In the more recent data from Cathedral City and Parkham Units shown in the exercises previously, you can see that Category X clients accounted for 19.7 per cent of all admissions for Cathedral City and 28.1 per cent of all admissions for Parkham Unit.

This has been found in other studies in 1994/1995 where the percentage has ranged from 10 per cent - 30 per cent of all admissions.

This raises a number of management issues. Apart from the costs involved and the disappointment for the clients who come into hospital expecting to deliver, only to return home and be readmitted at a later date, admitting these clients to the delivery suite means that midwives may be called away from women in labour in order to assess the Category X client. Such interruption adds to the stress of a busy suite, and might lead to the fragmentation of intrapartum care at a crucial moment.

The earlier study in Trent found that many of these clients were admitted to the wards by junior doctors, sometimes staying in for a number of days. Notional costs per month were allocated to this practice for midwife time, use of equipment at £50.00 per case where the woman was discharged after a short time on the delivery suite/antenatal ward and at £120.00 per case where the woman stayed overnight in a postnatal ward.

The estimated costs per month were very illuminating (Ball, 1992):

	Category X Number	Cost per month	
Unit		(£50) £	(£120) £
Unit A	121	6050	14520
Unit B	116	5800	13920
Unit C	243	121,502	29160
Unit D	93	4650	11160
Unit E	161	8050	19230
Unit F	169	8450	20280
Unit G	181	9050	21720

Solutions?

Obviously, some of these clients do need to come into hospital, either because of social isolation, distances to be travelled, transport issues, but many of them do not.

Some units have sought to solve this difficulty by providing a separate day unit for such admissions, and/or admitting them to the antenatal ward, rather than the delivery suite.

Others have determined admission screening policies which seek to prevent unnecessary admissions whilst still ensuring that any cases at risk are admitted and examined. It remains to be seen whether the advent of caseload based work, where the midwife is the first contact and visits her client at home will bring about a reduction of these admissions. Managers will need to consider how to handle this situation and whether their delivery suite has the capacity to admit these clients or not.

Using data for quality review

The case-mix distribution can provide useful information by which to measure outcomes of intrapartum care. As has been seen in our earlier case-studies, the score sheet itself can demonstrate how appropriate interventions in labour can produce good outcomes at delivery and for the baby.

Often the good outcome is overlooked in review processes which may focus only on the bad outcomes, and this is a pity. It is a useful exercise to look in detail at the normal deliveries who fall into the categories IV and V.

Looking at the overall data can also assist in quality review but this should be restricted in the main to comparing the units outcomes against its own targets or expectations. Caution should be exercised if comparing one's outcomes with that of another unit. There may be differences in the population which affect the results, or in the facilities available. If such a comparison is done as part of a quality exercise then the units to be compared should have similar numbers of births per annum and provide similar facilities such as neonatal care, operating theatre and epidural service.

Using data from controlled studies or evaluation of new care practices

Because the case-mix data encapsulates both process and outcome data, it can be very useful in controlled studies of different care policies within a unit. Perhaps comparing the outcomes of clients allocated to midwife managed care with a similar population in terms of risk factors who are allocated to the usual medical team led care.

The outcomes of different midwife teams can also be compared and used to produce individual team workload and staffing. Undertaking such studies can help to offset anxiety about change, and serve to highlight unexpected anomalies in workload distribution.

Summary

In this section we have explored the principles and application of *Birthrate* in intrapartum care and seen how it:

- captures the processes and outcome of labour

- records the mean midwife time needed to meet the client's need of care, and increases the percentage of midwife care in accordance to increased need of the client

- provides a formula for converting the data into staffing requirements, allowing for application of minimum or local allowances for holidays, sickness etc.

- produces a case-mix based upon process and outcome of labour which allows for comparisons of different care policies

- informs a number of management and quality issues.

UNIT FOUR

Using Case-Mix Data to Determine the Number of Beds Needed

In unit four we begin to use the Birthrate data with other local information to assess the number of beds required for local needs.

Section 4.1: Discusses the way that sound case-mix data provides a picture of local needs and patterns of care which affect resource needs.

Section 4.2: Describes how case-mix data can be used to assess the number of delivery suite beds needed.

Section 4.3: Discusses how case-mix data can be used to assess the number of postnatal beds in relation to the length of stay for women in the different outcome categories.

Section 4.4: Suggests a method for assessing the number of beds needed for antenatal care and Category X clients.

Section 4.5: Explores the difference which changes in length of stay makes to the number of beds required and uses as examples three hospitals of different sizes.

Section 4.1

The value of case-mix data

In the previous section, we saw how collecting *Birthrate* data provides a maternity service with case-mix information which encapsulates all the varying clinical and workload inducing factors which are involved in the labour and delivery of mothers and their infants.

The processes and outcomes of labour should be regarded as the fulcrum around which all other care needs revolve. Apart from a very small percentage of women who might develop some postnatal emergency after transfer from delivery suite, perhaps an unexpected haemorrhage, undetected trauma, or some crisis with the infant which was not apparent at birth, the pattern of postnatal care will be predetermined by the events of labour. Therefore the intrapartum case-mix provides a substantial basis for judging and planning the volume of postnatal care needed, both in hospital and community services.

The monthly and annual patterns of outcomes reflected in the *Birthrate* data have been found to be surprisingly consistent month by month, even though the daily patterns of work fluctuate considerably.

Birthrate data therefore reveals the patterns of need care practices provided by individual services for their local situation. This is a very important factor for managers seeking to accurately cost their services according to the demands made upon them and to assess the likely impact of changes in either workload or care policies. It also enables managers and clinicians to evaluate their current care patterns and assess whether these are both acceptable to their clients and effective in the use of resources.

As we continue through this manual, the question of local appraisal and decisions and policies will play a significant role in determining workforce needs.

How the section is structured

For each section we will first present the principle upon which staffing and bed calculations are made, and then explore variations which may be applied according to the local situation.

Section 4.2

Assessing the number of beds required

One of the main problems in assessing delivery suite beds is the unpredictability of the client needs at any one time.

The patterns of admission vary from day to day. Clients rarely follow each other consecutively and often most beds are full at one time of the day and empty for the rest. Therefore we have to build in some safeguards to allow for this.

Experience in using *Birthrate* indicates that the case-mix data, plus the mean length of time in delivery suite recorded per category, provides helpful information in making decisions about bed numbers, together with relevant local information.

Data to be used should span a minimum of six months in order to allow for most variations in care patterns, with annual data being the ideal basis.

It would seem simple to multiply the mean daily number of cases per category by the mean daily hours per category to produce the daily mean bed hours required. But women do not enter the ward in a sequential manner - some times most of the day's total number of clients will be in the labour ward at the same time, at others no more than three of four clients will be in the ward together.

However it should also be remembered that the mean hours per category illustrated in the table overleaf already include an increased percentage of time for Categories III - V and this will provide some extra lee-way for use of beds. However Categories IV and V may use both a labour bed and a separate delivery room during the course of their stay.

Another difficulty is that the daily number of cases per category is based upon the mean number of cases, and some days will be much higher and others much lower. Ideally one would use the mean and one standard deviation to calculate numbers per day, but many midwifery units do not have the facilities to do this.

Therefore, we have concluded that adding 30 per cent to daily mean number of cases per category and multiplying this figures by the mean hours per category provides a reasonable basis for assessing the number of beds needed. A further percentage allowance for bed occupancy can also be added if required.

In the example shown opposite we are using again the real data from Cathedral City Hospital which was shown in Section 7 of Unit 3 (p.52).

Cathedral City Hospital Annual Data

	BIRTHRATE CATEGORIES					
	I	II	III	IV	V	TOTAL
% Casemix	10.8	36.9	19.2	14.2	18.9	100
No cases p.a.	324	1107	576	426	567	3000
Daily mean no. cases	0.89	3.03	1.58	1.17	1.55	8.22
Mean hours per case	5.9	7.9	12.6	15.3	24.8	

Note: The mean hours per case is equal to the mean time in delivery suite recorded on the Birthrate records but with additional time added to Categories III - V to reflect increased midwife workload.

How to assess delivery bed needs

1.   Multiply the daily mean number of cases per category by 1.3 to increase it by 30 per cent.

2.   Multiply this figure by the daily mean hours per category (which includes the increase for Categories III-V) and total.

3.   Produce totals for 1 and 2 above which will give you the enhanced total of hours in the delivery suite for all categories.

4.   Divide the total hours in the delivery suite by 24 hours to produce the number of beds required per day and round up to a whole number.

Calculating the beds required

	BIRTHRATE CATEGORIES					
	I	II	III	IV	V	TOTAL
Daily mean no. cases	0.89	3.03	1.58	1.17	1.55	8.22
x 1.3 =	1.16	3.94	2.05	1.52	2.02	10.69
Mean hours per case	5.9	7.9	12.6	15.3	24.8	
Daily hours =	6.84	31.13	25.83	23.26	50.1	137.16

Divide the total daily hours by 24 hours =137.16 /24 = 5.72 beds needed which rounds up to six beds.

Now we need to add the beds for Category X, A and R cases. From the data given earlier we know that there were 736 Category X cases, 53 Category A and 35 Category R per annum, and the daily mean numbers were:

- Category X: 2.02 time allocated = 1 hour per case
- Category A: 0.15 with an average stay of 18.3 hours
- Category R: 0.1 with an average stay of 9 hours.

We do not need to plan for such a high degree of variability for these clients. We know that Category X cases need a short time for assessment and could be moved to an antenatal ward if needed, and that Category R cases are women returning after delivery for some extra emergency or planned treatment. But we do need to do so for Category A which are emergency admissions. Therefore we apply the same principle of adding 30 per cent to the number of Category A cases as we did for the delivered cases, but not for the others.

We assess beds needed as follows:

- Category X: 2.02 x 1   =   2.02 bed hours per day
- Category R: 0.1 x 9 hours   =   0.9 hours per day
- Category A: 0.15 x 18.3 x 1.3   =   3.57 hours per day

- Total daily bed hours   =   2.02 + 0.9 +3.57
                               =   6.49

- divide by 24 hours   =   6.49/24
                               =   0.27 beds

This total is added to that of the delivery beds.

In our example this would work out at: 5.72 + 0.27 = 5.99 beds which suggest that six beds would be sufficient. However, many managers might feel more confident at planning on six beds for deliveries and one more for other cases. A bed occupancy rate of 80 per cent would mean that 7.2 beds were needed.

Section 4.3

Assessing the number of postnatal beds required

The volume of postnatal beds required will depend upon two factors:

1. the volume and case-mix of mothers and babies
2. the usual or planned length of hospital postnatal stay in a particular service or population.

Both of these factors will be influenced by the needs of the population served and the care policies agreed between the purchaser and provider authorities, but cost implication should also be taken into consideration.

Large specialist units which cater for more complicated cases, including those transferred in labour from smaller units, have a larger percentage of cases in Categories III, IV and V, especially where there is an intensive neonatal unit.

Population and policy factors include consumer expectations of choice, social needs such as a significant number of families living in bed and breakfast accommodation, care policies which encourage a longer stay for primigravide or for mothers who live a large distance from the maternity unit or in isolated country areas.

Management dilemmas

Birthrate data from a wide variety of units and geographical locations indicate that the largest percentage of mothers (60 per cent or more) go home within 48 hours of delivery, and although this should be largely a question of consumer choice, (Cumberlege, 1993 pp.32-34; NHSME, 1993), there are cost implications if postnatal stay is extended unless there are clinical or social factors which make it desirable.

Early data from a major project evaluating the effectiveness of caseload management, and based on a sample of 1500 women (Page et al, 1995), indicates that women receiving care from midwives as the lead professional return home significantly earlier in the puerperium than do women receiving traditional hospital and community midwifery care.

These are all matters which call for local information and judgement and this should form part of the decision making process.

How to assess postnatal bed needs

1. Obtain the percentage case-mix from the *Birthrate* data
2. Estimate (from current or planned care-policies) the likely number of postnatal days in hospital required by mothers in the five *Birthrate* categories for delivered women
3. Decide the percentage bed occupancy you plan to work on.

Information which may help

Experience in many units indicates that almost all the women in Categories I, II and III go home within two or three days.

A study in 1993 (Washbrook) showed that 30 per cent of Category IV cases also go home on the third day, and further data based on 700 births in one unit and 400 in another showed that the most common time for women in Category IV to go home was on the fourth postnatal day (Washbrook, 1995).

This may seem surprising, but it should be remembered that most of the factors which allocate women to Category III and IV are labour related and transitory in their effects e.g. the most common factor which puts a woman in Category III is an epidural followed by episiotomy but with a normal delivery and healthy baby. The same is true for many in Category IV where a long labour, aided by an epidural and/or a forceps delivery but with a healthy outcome for the baby.

Where problems with the baby put a woman in a higher category, this will usually be Category IV and V.

In the case of a stillbirth however, (mercifully not a large number) the mother would be in Category IV or V but would usually want to return home as quickly as possible.

Women who have an elective caesarean section often go home around the fifth day whilst emergency caesarean section cases stay longer.

Many units have found it helpful to record length of stay against the *Birthrate* category to assist or confirm their decisions about length of stay.

Explanation of method

In the table shown, the process of calculation is:

1. Take *Birthrate* data on number and percentage of cases per category over the year.

2. Determine the likely number of postnatal days required for women in each category. This can be done in two ways; the most simple is to allocate an average length of stay per category, but where good information provides a break down of different lengths of stay within a category then that should be used.

For example, in many units a sizeable percentage of Category I clients go home on the day of delivery or within 24 hours, and this trend is likely to rise when caseload work teams have been established. Also as noted earlier, up to 30 per cent of Category IV cases go home on the third day. In the examples which follow we will first show the data in broad categories and then repeat it with split categories to show what difference is made when more specific data on length of stay is available.

The length of stay should reflect the number of bed days needed. Each bed day spans one midnight. Therefore if a woman delivers at 6.00 hours and goes home at 18.00 hours she has used one bed day, but if a woman delivers at 13.00 hours one day and goes home at 11.00 hours the next, then she has used two bed days, even though she has been in the ward for 23 hours.

3. Multiply the number of cases per category by the given number of bed days in the ward to determine the total bed days per annum e.g. Cat III: 576 women multiplied by 3 bed days = 1728 bed days.

4. Divide by 365 days to obtain the daily number of beds needed per category and add together to form total bed needs.

5. Add a percentage to this total which reflect variability of demand and the appropriate or required bed occupancy rate.

In the example shown opposite the added amount is 15 per cent which is equal to a bed occupancy rate of 85 per cent.

This is quite high, some units may wish to plan on 80 per cent bed occupancy, in which case you would add 20 per cent for variability.

Examples of assessing postnatal beds in different sized units

In the examples given we shall show two different sizes of units, and these will be used again when we calculate staffing needs for the ward. Later we will repeat the process with a third unit which has less than 2000 births per annum in order to explore the special staffing needs of small units.

Cathedral City Hospital

Assessing the number of postnatal beds needed for 3000 births per annum and annual *Birthrate* case-mix

BIRTHRATE CATEGORIES						
	I	II	III	IV	V	TOTAL
% Casemix	10.8	36.9	19.2	14.2	18.9	100
No cases p.a.	324	1107	576	426	567	3000
No days stay in ward	2	2	3	5	7	
No postnatal days p.a.	648	2214	1728	2130	3969	10689
/365 days p.a. = daily beds needed	1.78	6.07	4.7	5.84	10.87	29.28
Add 15% variability	2.04	7.0	5.4	6.7	12.5	33.68

The number of beds needed for this pattern of need = **33.68 beds**.

If the planned bed occupancy was 80 per cent then 20 per cent would be added to the total at stage 4; **29.28 x 1.2 = 35.14 beds**.

Now we need to calculate the beds needed on the wards for antenatal care, Category X etc.

Section 4.4

Calculating beds for Category X clients and antenatal care

Principle:

1. Determine what percentage of Category X are likely to be admitted to the ward. Managers may decide to admit all Category X to the ward rather than the delivery suite, in which case you would use the total per annum shown. Or they may decide to admit to the delivery suite but send them home from there, rather than admit them for a further stay on the ward.

2. Multiply the number by two bed days to produce total bed days required.

3. Add percentage for bed occupancy as for postnatal beds.

Cathedral City hospital:

In this hospital the annual number of Category X admissions to the delivery suite equals 736 (24.5 per cent of all admissions). In the past, whether or not a woman was admitted to the ward was dependent on the decision of the junior doctor on duty at the time, and it is not known how many were admitted to the ward or how many went home direct from the delivery suite.

Decisions made

A number of decisions have now been made to reduce the workload created by Category X's and it is hoped to reduce admissions as a whole by 10 per cent, which means that the manager expects Category X to be 15.5 per cent of 3000 admissions per year equalling 465 cases, and that only 40 per cent of these (186) will be kept admitted to the ward. As these are often overnight, then two bed days are involved.

- 186 x 2 bed days = 372 bed days per annum
- Divide by 365 = 1.02 beds + 15 per cent
  = **1.17 beds**.

Calculating for antenatal beds

To calculate the number of beds for antenatal care:

1. Assess or estimate what number are admitted per annum remembering to exclude Category X cases who would normally be admitted from the delivery suite.

2. Assess or estimate how many of these are low risk/short stay for induction/ monitoring and how many are high risk needing a longer stay (pregnancy induced hypertension, antepartum haemorrhage, threatened premature birth etc.)

In the absence of detailed records on antenatal care, most units assume that 70 per cent will be low risk needing one or two bed days and 30 per cent will be high risk staying an average of five bed days per patient episode.

3. Add percentage for bed occupancy.

In the example given for Cathedral City, antenatal admissions are estimated at 20 per cent of all births which equals 600 cases per annum.

To calculate bed days needed:

- 70 per cent = 420 x 1.5 bed days = 630 bed days
- 30 per cent = 180 x 5 bed days = 900 bed days
- total bed days = 1530/365
  = 4.19 bed days + 15%
  = **4.82**

- Total ward beds required = **33.68** p/natal
  + 1.17 Category X + 4.82 antenatal = **39.67 beds**

Therefore = **40 beds** are needed.

Section 4.5

Effect on changes in the length of stay

Now we will repeat the exercise but this time the length of stay for some categories will be split.

Cathedral City Hospital

Assessing the number of postnatal beds needed for 3000 births per annum and annual *Birthrate* case-mix

BIRTHRATE CATEGORIES						
	I	II	III	IV	V	TOTAL
% Casemix	10.8	36.9	19.2	14.2	18.9	100
No cases p.a.	324	1107	576	426	567	3000

This time the length of stay is calculated at:

- Category I: 10 per cent =   32 cases x 1 day =   32 bed days
-              90 per cent = 292 cases x 2 days =   584 bed days
- Category II   = 1107 cases x 2 bed days = 2214 bed days
- Category III   = 576 cases x 3 bed days = 1728 bed days
- Category IV: 30 per cent = 128 cases x 3 bed days =   384 bed days
-              70 per cent = 298 cases x 5 bed days = 1490 bed days
- Category V: 20 per cent = 113 cases x 5 bed days =   565 bed days
-              80 per cent = 454 cases x 7 bed days = 3178 bed days

    TOTAL   = 10175 bed days

So now we have a total of 10175 bed days per annum which is a reduction of 514 on previous calculation. If we add:

- 15 per cent for variation and bed occupancy =   11701 bed days
- and *divide* by 365 days   =   **32.06 beds** needed

If we add the same number of beds as before for antenatal and Category X cases equalling **5.99**, then the total beds needed are **38.05**, which means we could plan on 38 beds rather than 40 previously calculated. Although this does not seem to be a large saving, the difference made by splitting the time allocation in certain categories will also make a difference in staffing requirements.

The next example is of a larger unit with 5250 births a year, and an increased percentage of cases in the higher categories.

Majorport Hospital
Assessing the number of postnatal beds needed for 5250 births per annum and annual *Birthrate* case-mix

	\multicolumn{6}{c}{**BIRTHRATE CATEGORIES**}
	I	II	III	IV	V	TOTAL
% Casemix	13.1	18.0	23.4	21.9	23.6	100
No cases p.a.	687	946	1230	1150	1237	5250
No of days stay in ward	2	2	3	5	7	
No postnatal days p.a.	1374	1892	3690	5750	8659	21365
/365 days p.a. = daily beds needed	3.8	5.2	10.1	15.8	23.7	58.53
Add 15% for variability	4.4	6.0	11.6	18.2	27.3	67.3

You can see in this and in Cathedral City data how the bulk of the bed needs is for complicated cases.

On this basis we need **67.3 beds** for postnatal care.

Add bed days for Category X and antenatal cases.

If Category X = 20 per cent of all admissions (=1050 per annum and 40 per cent = 420) are admitted to the ward, then we need:

$$420 \times 2 = 840/365 \quad = 2.30 \times 1.15 \quad = \quad \textbf{2.65 beds}.$$

There may be more antenatal admissions in a large unit like this, especially with its neonatal services. It is estimated that 30 per cent of all admissions are antenatal with 60 per cent short stay and 40 per cent long stay:

- Total antenatal admissions per annum = 1575

    60 per cent of these are short stay = 945 at 1.5 bed days each
    = 1417.5/365
    = 3.88 x 1.15
    = 4.47 beds
    40 per cent = 630 x 5 days = 3150/365
    = 8.63 x 1.15
    = 9.92 beds

    Total antenatal beds needed **= 14.39**

Total number of beds based on 5250 births per annum, the case-mix and length of stay shown by the local situation and at planned 85 per cent occupancy:

- 67.3 postnatal
- 2.65 Category X
- 14.39 antenatal =

- **84.34** so plan on **84 beds**.

What would be the effect of splitting lengths of stay per category in this unit?

If we applied to this unit the split lengths of stay which were used in the second version of Cathedral City then the bed needs would be as follows:

- Category I (687): 10 per cent = 69 cases x 1 day = 69 bed days
    90 per cent = 618 cases x 2 days = 1236 bed days
- Category II = 946 x 2 bed days = 1892 bed days
- Category III = 1230 x 3 bed days = 3690 bed days
- Category IV: 30 per cent = 345 x 3 bed days = 1035 bed days
    70 per cent = 805 x 5 bed days = 4025 bed days
- Category V: 20 per cent = 247 x 5 bed days = 1237 bed days
    80 per cent = 990 x 7 bed days = 6927 bed days

- Total beds days needed = 20111/365 + 15 per cent
    = 63.36 beds

    add 2.65 and 14.39 beds for antenatals **= 80.35 beds**

Plan on **80 beds**, which is a reduction of **4 beds**.

In summary of the two units, Cathedral City and Majorport Hospital, it can be seen that the larger the number of births per annum the greater the difference which can be made if specific lengths of stay can be used to assess bed needs.

Planning for small units

The next example is based on real data from a small unit, which caters for women across a large area of beautiful countryside but with twisting, and in the summer, congested roads. You will see a different case-mix with the largest percentage in Category II and a longer length of stay in Categories II and III which reflects local choices for the early postnatal days, but lesser stays for the other categories.

Lakeside Hospital

Assessing the number of postnatal beds needed for 1500 births per annum and annual *Birthrate* case-mix

BIRTHRATE CATEGORIES						
	I	II	III	IV	V	TOTAL
% Casemix	13.3	41.6	17.8	14.9	12.4	100
No cases p.a.	200	624	267	223	186	1500
No of days stay in ward	2	3	4	5	6	
No postnatal days p.a.	400	1872	1068	1115	1116	15183
/365 days p.a. = daily beds needed	1.1	5.13	2.93	3.05	3.06	15.27
Add 15%* for variability	1.3	5.9	3.37	3.51	3.52	17.6

Different patterns in small units

On the data shown above **17.6 beds** are needed for postnatal care, but it is very unlikely that such a small unit could achieve 85 per cent bed occupancy. It would be wiser to plan on 70 per cent bed occupancy which would require 19.85 beds (15.27 + 30 per cent = **15.27 x 1.3 = 19.85**).

Category X and antenatal cases

Secondly, a rural unit like this is likely to have a higher percentage of Category X cases, as women are more likely to come in where they live a considerable distance from the unit. For the same reason they are likely to be kept in just in case labour commences.

The actual data for this unit was that Category X equalled 33 per cent of all admissions, and it is not likely that this can be reduced to any degree before Cumberlege type midwife work has been established.

Beds needed for Category X therefore:

- = 33 per cent of 1500   = 495 cases per annum

- if 50 per cent stay overnight in the ward:
  = 248 x 2 bed days   = 496/365 = 1.02 + 30%
  = 1.77 beds

ANTENATAL

There will be fewer long stay antenatal cases as any serious complications are likely to be transferred to a larger unit, and the real data for all antenatal admissions equals 84 per annum.

If 80 per cent are short stay:

- 80 per cent of 84   =   67 cases x 1.5 days
                           =   100.5 per annum
  divide by 365 days   =   0.28 bed days

  20 per cent of 84   =   17 x 5 bed days
                           =   85 per annum
  divide by 365   =   0.23 bed days

- Total
  0.23 + 0.28   =   0.51 bed days
  + 30 per cent bed occupancy =   0.51 x 1.13
                           =   **0.67 beds**

Total beds needed for 1500 births, different length of stay, more Category X, fewer long stay antenatals and at 30 per cent bed occupancy.

- =   19.85 + 1.77 + 0.66
- =   22.28 bed days; plan on **22** beds.

Differences in need required by local situations

PLANNING CARE AND BUDGETS FOR SERVICES

The examples given above highlight the importance of local factors and decisions in deciding the resources required, but also show how such factors can be clearly identified in local care contracts, so that appropriate costings can be produced.

These differences in the resources required will also be seen in the following calculations of staffing needs on the wards and in the community services, and we will be looking again at safeguards which need to be built into staffing levels for small units.

Being able to clearly identify resource needs is particularly important when decisions are being made about possible developments of the service, such as implementation of Cumberlege or when other changes such as an increase in births, or merger with maternity services etc. are being envisaged.

UNIT FIVE

Using Case-Mix Data as a Basis for Calculating Ward Staffing Needs

In this unit we will use the case-mix data as before, but this time we will add local decisions of length of stay and midwife hours per category.

This unit will complete the staffing calculations for a total hospital.

Section 5.1: Explains the principles for assessing midwife hours per category for postnatal care by consensus.

Section 5.2: Explains how to calculate staffing numbers for postnatal care and introduces midwife hours per annum as the basis for turning total hours into whole-time equivalents.

Section 5.3: Explains how to calculate staff for Category X and antenatal cases.

Section 5.4: Discusses the impact of shorter lengths of stay upon ward staffing need and introduces the issue of option appraisal.

Section 5.5: Discusses how to use shift patterns and local decisions to determine the number of health care assistants needed for the wards.

Section 5.6: Looks at the special situation for small units and the need to add staff above workload calculations to ensure safety across 24 hours of care.

Section 5.7: Suggests a framework for calculating staff needed to run hospital based clinics and parentcraft sessions.

Section 5.8: Provides a summary of the work undertaken in Units Four and Five and shows a staffing profile completed for the hospital services for Cathedral City Hospital which has been produced as we have worked out the examples in Units Three, Four and Five.

Section 5.1

Assessing staffing needs for the ward areas

This process follows closely on that shown previously for assessing the beds required. As before we will need to know:

1.   the volume and case-mix of mothers and babies
2.   the usual length of hospital postnatal stay in a particular locality
3.   some assessment of the amount of midwife time per day required by mothers in the different *Birthrate* categories.

Estimating midwife time for postnatal care

Here lies something of a dilemma. It would be possible to assess the midwife time needed per *Birthrate* category by non-participant observation, but this would be a very costly process. It would be necessary to gain such data over 24 hours a day, and for at least a month in order to capture sufficient data to reflect typical patterns of care in an area where the pattern of admissions can fluctuate considerably day by day, and where client need can also vary in intensity. There would also need to be some measure of quality of care if one is to avoid measuring midwife time, which is either insufficient for client need, or where midwife time is not used effectively and efficiently.

Research has shown that there are considerable problems in gaining accurate activity data, especially where staff record their own activity and time spent on various aspects of patient care (Hurst, 1993 pp.77-78).

Midwifery is perhaps in a more fortunate position than nursing in this area because our population is confined to healthy women between the ages of 14 - 45 years, the *Birthrate* category already classifies the clients according to labour outcome and the length of postnatal care is well defined in the literature.

For these practical and methodological reasons, units using *Birthrate* have produced estimated midwife time per patient category day by professional judgement, debate and consensus. The midwife time per category day includes all direct and indirect care of the client and baby by midwives, and clients will also receive care from health care assistants. Just as was done for delivery suite staffing, 15 per cent is added to allow for fluctuation in workload, co-ordination of care between agencies, and other associated work, and a further five per cent is also added for management, co-ordination, teaching and staff meetings during postnatal care.

Therefore the midwife times produced by this method are based on the premise that 80 per cent of midwife time is spent on direct and indirect care of clients with 20 per cent allowed for co-ordination, meetings etc, and with health care assistants providing the bulk of associated work (see below).

This compares with the percentages of 65 per cent direct and indirect nursing care and 24 per cent associated work by trained nurses identified by activity analysis in 17 medical wards which were meeting required quality standards (Hurst, 1993).

Basis for estimated midwife hours

The midwife hours per category day produced by these consensus discussions are explained below. Midwife managers will know their own unit's policies on postnatal stay and can apply the appropriate pattern. However, because there are anomalies in how length of stay is discussed in hospital, the same criteria should be applied as for assessing beds i.e. if a woman stays overnight she has used two bed days. In many maternity units a custom has arisen of assuming that 12.00 hours marks the difference between the various postnatal days, so that a woman delivered before 12.00 hours has that day counted as her 'first' day but one delivered at 13.00 hours does not, a situation not appreciated by clients!

On the basis of numerous discussions and assessments of staff needs therefore, we would recommend the following guidelines on midwife time required. It is perhaps important to remind readers that the time allocated on day one will be in addition to the time already spent on the delivery suite, and that given for the day of discharge assumes that the mother and baby usually leave in the morning or before 16.00 hours.

Estimated midwife hours per category stay
It is important to point out that the midwife time shown below is based upon the premise that midwives are primarily caring for their clients, with health care assistants (who will be discussed later) assisting midwives, providing all housekeeping and family type care to mothers and babies, together with some routine clerical work.

Categories I and II (the most normal labour and delivery)

If the mother is delivered one day and discharged the next, the input is two hours per day. If however the mother is discharged on the third day, then the input is two hours for the first and third day, three hours for the second day. If the mother is discharged on the same day as delivery then two hours seems reasonable to add to the time already spent on the delivery suite.

Category III

These are usually discharged on the third postnatal day. Time is assessed as four hours on day one because mother may require a good deal of help with the baby, be less active after epidural/forceps/long labour, three hours on the second day and another two hours on the day of discharge.

Category IV

Now there are more variables to deal with as numerous factors might put a woman and baby into Categories IV and V. The mother may have had a traumatic labour and/ or delivery, she may have a sick or premature baby. Discussion with a number of units indicates that the most frequent length of stay is five days, and a study in 1993 (Washbrook) showed that approximately 30 per cent of Category IV cases go home on the third day.

Therefore the assessment is as follows:

The general consensus on midwife time per Category day has been as follows:

- Day 1   6.0 hours
- Day 2   5.0 hours
- Day 3   4.5 hours
- Day 4   3.0 hours
- Day 5   2.0 hours   (if this is the day of discharge, if not 3.0 hours per day until the day of discharge when two hours is allocated).

Category V

This category has a similar pattern but as this is the one where the mother will have been most in need during labour, and includes caesarean sections, and any multiple births, then midwives will need to care for the baby as well as the mother, for some time before the mother is able to cope. Therefore, the assessment is:

- Days 1 and 2   7.0 hours per day
- Day 3   6.0 hours
- Day 4   5.0 hours
- Day 5   4.0 hours
- Day 6   3.0 hours   (with two hours on the day of discharge which may be on Day 5, 6 or later according to degree of need).

The midwife time per Category day discussed above is shown in the following grid, so that the total midwife time per Category stay can be assessed on the basis of the number of days stay for different categories determined by local care policies.

In each case, the last day shown is the day of discharge. In units, where the stay is normally longer than that shown, appropriate adjustments should be made.

Midwife managers are of course free to produce their own estimated times per Category, but are warned that there are dangers in applying excessive midwife hours per day and this will be shown in larger than expected or reasonable staffing numbers. Adjustments for the special needs of small units will be discussed later in this chapter.

Midwife hours per Birthrate category and local length of stay

DAYS IN WARD	I	II	III	IV	V
Day 1	2	2	4	6	7
Day 2	2	2	3	5	7
Day 3			2	4.5	6
Day 4				3	5
Day 5				2	4
Day 6					3
Day 7					2
TOTALS	4*	4*	9	20.5	34

How to use the grid

Assess what your patterns are and multiply the days by the appropriate hours.

* There may be variation in the length of stay in these groups e.g. if most Category I's go home after one night in hospital then use the figures above. If they go home after two nights in hospital then use three hours for the middle day. If they go home on the same day as delivery then use first day hours only. The same applies to Category II cases.

If Category IV cases go home on the sixth, then add another three hours to the total for this group of women = 23.5 hours.

Section 5.2

Calculating midwife time for postnatal care in hospital

Unlike the delivery suite, we shall base the staffing numbers on annual hours needed.

Allowances of 15 per cent variability and five per cent management will be added as before, and the total midwife hours will be divided by 1612.5 hours per annum.

Why 1612.5 hours per annum?

This figure is based upon the current national holiday allowances and a minimum of two weeks for sickness and study leave. However, different annual hours should be applied where managers consider that two weeks sickness is too small an allowance or where health authorities or trusts have produced their own sickness allowances and/or holiday entitlement.

The details of how these figures are calculated are shown below.

1. **Based on current holiday entitlement and a minimum estimate of sickness etc.**

    52 weeks per annum:
    Deduct   7 weeks holiday (5 weeks annual leave + 10 bank holidays)

    Deduct   a minimum allowance of **2 weeks sickness and/or study leave**

    Total =   9 weeks (= 17.3 per cent of total 52 weeks)

    52 - 9 = 43 weeks x 37.5 hours per week = **1612.5** hours per annum per w.t.e. midwife.

This would reflect total establishment needs.

In post staffing figures:
    52 weeks x 37.5 = 1950 midwife hours per annum.

2.   Based on agreed local terms and sickness rates

In many units different rates apply. If this is the case in a local situation, then the local allowance should be used to calculate annual hours.

e.g.   **3** weeks sickness plus holidays   = 52 - 10 weeks
                                                = 42 x 37.5
                                                = **1575** midwife hours per annum
                                                (19.2 per cent allowance)

          4 weeks sickness plus holidays   = 52 - 11 weeks
                                                = 41 x 37.5
                                                = **1537.5** midwife hours per annum
                                                (21.2 per cent allowance)

          5 weeks sickness plus holidays   = 52 - 12 weeks
                                                = 40 x 37.5
                                                = **1500** midwife hours per annum
                                                (23.0 per cent allowance)

It is perhaps surprising to see what a difference is made by different allowances for holidays and sickness.

Nevertheless, local conditions and care practices do need to be taken into consideration when assessing staffing needs.

Managers should apply their own level of annual hours in relation to local policies. If none exist then we suggest that one of the figures shown in 1 or 2 above should be applied.

For the examples used in this manual, we will be using 1612.5 as the total midwife hours per annum. This represents the lowest feasible allowances.

Examples of calculating staff needed for ward areas

In the examples given overleaf, we will use Cathedral City Hospital and use two different amounts of postnatal stay, shown earlier, to demonstrate the impact that small differences in care patterns can have on staffing numbers.

Cathedral City Hospital

Assessing the ward based staffing needs based on 3000 births per annum and annual *Birthrate* case-mix

BIRTHRATE CATEGORIES						
	I	II	III	IV	V	TOTAL
No days stay in ward	2	2	3	5	7	
% casemix	10.8	36.9	19.2	14.2	18.9	100
No case p.a.	324	1107	576	426	567	3000
Midwife hours per stay	4	4	9	20.5	34	
Total Midwife hrs p.a.	1296	4428	5184	8733	19278	38919

Total midwife hours per annum for all direct and indirect care:

- = 38919 hours per annum   *Add 15 per cent variability*

- = 38919 x 1.15

- = 44756.85 hours   *Add 5 per cent management etc.*

- = 44756.85 x 1.05

- = 46994.7 hours per annum

However we still need to calculate the staff needed for Category X and antenatal cases before we reach our final staffing establishment (see opposite).

Section 5.3

Category X and antenatal cases

In our earlier example with Cathedral City Hospital we saw that they had planned for 465 Category X cases staying two days on the ward and that there were 600 antenatals of which 420 were low risk, mainly for overnight induction and were assessed as needing 1.5 days stay. The other 180 were high risk staying five days.

The estimate of hours per day required by these cases is:

- Category X - 2 hours
- Low risk antenatal - 2 hours
- High risk antenatal - 3 hours per day.

To establish this figure multiply days in ward (No. 2) x Midwife hours per day (No.3)

	Antenatal low risk	Antenatal high risk	Category X	Total
1. No cases =	420	180	465	1065
2. Days in ward	1.5	5.0	2.0	
3. Midwife hours per day	2	3	2	
4. Midwife hours per stay	3	15	4	
TOTAL HOURS	1260	2700	1860	5820

5820 hours are needed for Category X and antenatal cases.

Because these cases are more predictable and admissions can generally be controlled we do not add 15 per cent for variability as in the delivery suite or postnatal care, but we do add the five per cent for management = 5820 x 1.05 = 6111 hours per annum.

Total midwife hours for all ward work

- 46994.7 postnatal *and*
- 6111.0 antenatal care
- 53105.7 hours of midwife time per annum.

The total midwife hours per annum is divided by 1612.5 hours to calculate the number of w.t.e. midwives needed for total funded establishment.

- = 53105.7/1612.5
- = **32.93 (33) w.t.e. midwives for all ward based work**

If there are two wards, then there are 16.5 w.t.e. midwives per ward.

Section 5.4

What is the impact of reducing the length of stay?

In the next example we will use the same number and case-mix of cases in Cathedral City Hospital, but use the different lengths of stay to produce staffing numbers.

Cathedral City Hospital (using second length of stay)
Assessing the staffing needs for ward based work 3000 births per annum and annual *Birthrate* case-mix

BIRTHRATE CATEGORIES						
	I	II	III	IV	V	Total
% Case-mix	10.8	36.9	19.2	14.2	18.9	100
No cases p.a.	324	1107	576	426	567	3000

This time the length of stay is calculated at:

- Category I: 10 per cent = 32 cases stay 1 day
  90 per cent = 292 cases stay 2 days
- Category II unchanged
- Category III unchanged
- Category IV: 30 per cent = 128 cases go home on third day
  70 per cent = 298 cases stay for 5 days
- Category V: 20 per cent = 113 go home on 5th day *and*
  80 per cent = 454 go home on 7th day

With these adjustments regarding the length of stay the number of midwife hours shown by the grid is applied.

e.g. 32 Category I will have 2 hours midwife time
128 Category IV will have 13 hours of midwife time - i.e.
Day 1 - 6 hrs
Day 2 - 5 hrs
Day 3 - 2 hrs (day of discharge).

Birthrate categories
Midwife hours needed per day

DAYS IN WARD	I	II	III	IV	V
Day 1	2	2	4	6	7
Day 2	2	2	3	5	7
Day 3			2	4.5	6
Day 4				3	5
Day 5				2	4
Day 6					3
Day 7					2
TOTALS	4*	4*	9	20.5	34

Midwife hours per stay

- Category I: 32 x 2 hours and 292 x 4 hours   = 1232 hours
- Category II: 1107 x 4 hours   = 4428 hours
- Category III: 576 x 9 hours   = 5184 hours
- Category IV: 128 x 13 hours   = 1664 hours
  -      298 x 20.5 hours   = 6109 hours
- Category V: 113 x 27 hours   = 3051 hours
  -      454 x 34 hours   = 15436 hours

Total midwife hours on this care pattern   = 37104.0 x 1.15
     = 42669.6 x 1.05

which is a reduction of **2191.62** hours per annum.

If this is divided by **1612.5**, it means a reduction of **1.4 w.t.e.** midwives.

This can be confirmed by adding the same totals as before for Category X and antenatal care on the wards:

     44803.08 + 6111 = 50914.08 = **31.6 w.t.e.** rather than the **32.93 w.t.e.** midwives.

But is it the 'right' answer? Only local knowledge and needs can determine that.

What checks and balances are needed to ensure adequate cover for 24 hours a day?

Option appraisal: using the 'what if...?' approach to plan staffing
The examples shown above in Cathedral City Hospital illustrate a difference can be made when care patterns or local guidelines on sickness and study leave are changed. This can be useful to a manager who may be faced with the need or demand to reduce her costs, but who fears that the quality of the service may be jeopardized if she does.

The mechanism shown illustrates how the case-mix and numbers of clients can be applied to a series of care/midwife input options to assess the number of staff needed for each. This gives some degree of control and opportunities for forward planning of services in line with available resources; alternatively it can be used to demonstrate the potential effect on client care standards if the funded establishment is below that shown to be essential.

Impact on community services

While it is important to ensure efficient use of hospital based resources, it is also important to remember that the postnatal care of a client does not end when she leaves the hospital but is continued by the community midwife.

Which option?

The manager therefore must assess which option provides the best answer to meeting the targets of providing effective, acceptable and efficient care patterns for the population being served.

For example, if in Cathedral City Hospital, the funded establishment for the wards is 30 w.t.e. midwives but the first criteria on length of stay were in force, which needs 32.93 w.t.e. then the manager would need to:

a)   review the basis for length of stay, and reduce it where possible, thus reducing demand to fit with capacity, or

b)   transfer extra staff, (if any were available) from another part of the service

c)   use the information from *Birthrate* to put her argument for an increase in staffing.

What would not be acceptable would be to leave the situation as it was.

Section 5.5

Adding health care assistants to the staff needed on wards

As noted previously, the midwife hours per Category day/stay are based on the premise that midwives will concentrate on providing direct and indirect care, with HCA's or Maternity Auxiliaries providing some direct care and dealing with all the associated work of providing a comfortable and safe environment.

The number of HCA's can be calculated by determining how many are needed per day as shown in the example below:

How many w.t.e. HCA's are needed?

Day shift	7.5 hours x 7 days	= 52.5 hours + 17.3% hols, = 61.58 hours /37.5 = 1.64 w.t.e.
Night shift	10 hours x 7 nights	= 70.00 + 17.3% = 82.11/37.5 = 2.2 w.t.e.

Therefore:

- 3 HCA's per shift on day duty
  3 x 2 shifts x 1.64 w.t.e.   = 9.84 w.t.e.

- 2 HCA's per shift on nights
  2 x 2.2 w.t.e.   = 4.4 w.t.e.

- Establishment needed   = 14.24 w.t.e.

Section 5.6

Special needs of small units

The need to demonstrate the linkage between staff numbers and care standards is dealt with further as we consider the special needs of small maternity units.

What is a 'small unit'?

Earlier research in nursing (Ball et al, 1989; Audit Commission, 1992) found that in wards with a smaller volume of workload, workload based staffing numbers would not be sufficient to staff the ward for 24 hours a day. The same has been found to be true in *Birthrate* studies.

Generally units caring for less than 2500 births per annum fall into this category.

In some general hospital wards, this problem can be resolved by converting much of the work to day cases, or closing wards at the weekend. In other situations e.g. a single acute paediatric ward, there is need to provide a 24 hour service of skilled children's nurses irrespective of the workload. Midwifery units are in a similar position as they generally provide the only maternity care service for a given geographical area.

Calculating the staff required over and above workload needs

This problem can be addressed by comparing the staffing produced by the workload measurement system with the numbers of staff required to run a service and fulfil duty of care to clients for 24 hours a day and seven days a week.

Principles

1. Calculate workforce based staffing needs

2. Decide how many midwives and HCA's are needed by shift to maintain effective care.

Taking the local shift pattern as the basis, work out the hours accounted for by the length of the shift and time for hand over between shifts. e.g.

	Midwives per shift day/night	Hours worked
Day shifts	7.00 - 15.00	8 hour span
	13.30 - 21.30	8 hour span
Night shift	21.00 - 7.30	10 hour span
		26 hour span over 24 hours

The spans shown above allow for meal breaks and an hour hand over at the end of the shift, plus some overlap on day duty.

The total span of 26 hours reflects total staff time over 24 hours. In many units, other shifts are worked and the overlap has been eliminated. The example shown above is intended simply to show the method.

Calculate establishment for one midwife per shift as follows:

Day shift	8 hours x 7 days	= 56 hours +17.3% hols, sickness, *etc* = 65.69 hours/37.5 = 1.75 w.t.e.
Night shift	10 hours x 7 nights	= 70 hours + 17.3% hols, sickness, *etc* = 82.1/37.5 = 2.2 w.t.e.

Determine the numbers of staff required per shift and multiply by the w.t.e. shown above.

WARD BASED WORK

e.g. 3 midwives per shift on day duty x 2 day shifts

$$= \quad 6 \times 1.75 \text{ w.t.e.}$$
$$= \quad 10.5 \text{ w.t.e.}$$

2 midwives per shift on night duty in a ward

$$= \quad 2 \times 2.2 \text{ w.t.e.}$$
$$= \quad 4.4 \text{ w.t.e.}$$

Minimum total staff by shift   =   *14.9 w.t.e*

DELIVERY SUITE

As clients are admitted and are in labour at any time of the day or night, then equal numbers of midwives are needed on each shift e.g. if four midwives per shift are considered essential on the delivery suite then the figures are:

Day shifts	4 morning x 1.75	= 7.0 w.t.e.
	4 late x 1.75	= 7.0 w.t.e.
Night shift	4 x 2.2	= 8.8 w.t.e.
Total		= 22.8 w.t.e.

- 3 midwives per shift   = 17.1 w.t.e.
- 4 midwives per shift   = 22.8 w.t.e.
- 5 midwives per shift   = 28.5 w.t.e.

Health care assistants should be added to ward and delivery suite as shown earlier.

Example from Lakeside Unit

If we use the previous data for Lakeside Hospital, we can demonstrate the decisions that need to be made.

The first example will be in detail and for ward staffing, followed by a resume of the delivery suite staffing needs.

You will remember that Categories II and III stayed longer than in Cathedral City, and Category V went home on the sixth day.

So midwife hours for   Category II = 7 hours,
Category III = 12 hours *and*
Category V = 31 hours.

Lakeside hospital

Assessing the number of midwives for wards based on 1500 births per annum and annual Birthrate case-mix.

BIRTHRATE CATEGORIES						
	I	II	III	IV	V	TOTAL
% casemix *	13.3	41.6	17.8	14.9	12.4	100
No cases p.a.	200	624	267	223	186	1500
No days stay in ward	2	3	4	5	6	
Midwife hours per total stay	4	7	12	20.5	31	
TOTAL HOURS	800	4368	3204	4571.5	5766	18709.5

Total midwife hours per annum for all direct and indirect postnatal care:

> = 18709.5 hours per annum   *Add 15 per cent variability*
> = 18709.5 x 1.15
> = 21515.93 hours + *5 per cent management etc*
> = 21515.93 x 1.05
> = *22591.72 hours per annum*

Now we need to add the hours for Category X and antenatal cases:

- Category X: = 248 stay overnight on ward
  - = 2 bed days x 2 midwife hours per day
  - = *992* hours

- Antenatals: = 84 per annum.

  If 80 per cent are short stay:
  - = 67 cases x 2 days x 2 midwife hours per day
  - = *268* hours

  20 per cent are long stay:
  - = 17 cases x 5 days x 3 midwife hours per day
  - = *255* hours

Total for X and antenatal care
> = *1515 hours*

Total midwife hours for all cases
> = 22591.72 + 1515
> = 24106.72 midwife hours per annum /1612.5
> = **14.95 w.t.e. midwives**

Check that this will provide safe numbers of midwives per shift.

We know that, on the basis of the shift pattern shown above, deploying three midwives per day shift and two per night shift required 14.9 w.t.e. This means that the workload based staffing needs match the minimum needed by shift allocation.

Now we will look at the delivery suite needs in Lakeside.

Lakeside hospital
Assessing the number of midwives needed for delivery suite based on 1500 births per annum and *Birthrate* case-mix

	BIRTHRATE CATEGORIES					
	I	II	III	IV	V	TOTAL
% casemix	13.3	41.6	17.8	14.9	12.4	100
No cases p.a.	200	624	267	223	186	1500
Daily mean =	.55	1.71	.73	.61	.51	4.11
Workload ratios	1.0	1.48	2.56	3.24	5.48	
Workload index	.55	2.53	1.87	1.98	2.79	9.72

Staffing formula:
Workload index   =   9.72
Midwife hours per Category I   =   5.02

Daily workload   =   9.72 x 5.02 = 48.79

Weekly workload   =   48.79 x 7
                              =   341.53 hours of m/w time
     +15% variance   =   392.75
     + 5% management, *etc*   =   412.39 hours /37.5
     In post   =   10.99 w.t.e.   (11 w.t.e.)
     add 17.3% holidays, *etc*   =   12.9 w.t.e.
     Establishment needed   **= 12.9 w.t.e.**

Now we have a dilemma:

This figure is less than that needed for three midwives per day shift and two per night shift, and we have already noted that equal numbers of staff are needed day and night in delivery suite.

If the manager staffs it at three midwives per shift (which is a very small margin for peaks of workload *or* sickness levels) then she needs:

-     3 x 1.75 x 2 day shifts   = 10.5 w.t.e.
-     3 x 2.2 per night shift   = 6.6. w.t.e.

Total = **17.1 w.t.e.** which is four more than needed by workload.

Some of this extra staff may be taken up by staffing needs for Category X, A and R.

These data show that there were:
- 496 Category X cases
- 65 Category A and
- 10 Category R cases per annum.

In addition there were:
- 15 escorts and
- 10 flying squad calls.

WORKLOAD BASED ON CATEGORY X, A, R AND OTHER WORK

- Category X: 496 x 1 hour   = 496 hours per annum
- Category A: 65 x 3.5 hours per case   = 227.5 hours
- Category R: 10 x 4.3 hours per case   = 43.0 hours
- 15 escorts x 1 midwife x 5.3 hours   = 79.5 hours
- 10 flying squad calls x 2 midwives   = 76 hours
- x 3.8 hours per call

- Total hours for this extra workload   = 922 hours per annum

- 922/52 weeks   = 17.73 hours per week
- + 15 per cent   = 20.39
                                               = 0.54 in post
- + 17.3 per cent   = 0.63 w.t.e. establishment

- *Total staff* for delivery suite   = 12.9 + 0.63
                                               = *13.53 w.t.e.*

Decisions: workload requires **13.5 w.t.e.** but minimum staffing levels need **17.1 w.t.e.**

Lakeside unit provides the maternity service for a large rural area, transferring complicated cases to a major unit some distance away. It would be unwise to staff the delivery suite with less than 17.1 w.t.e. as there is very little extra staff available on the wards in case of high workload or flying squad calls.

The manager may decide that there is need to fund up to four midwives per shift for delivery suite (22.8 w.t.e.) in order to ensure maximum flexibility. In which case, any staff needed for antenatal clinics etc will be drawn from that total.

Why do workload studies in small units?

In view of all this, it might be thought that there is little point in doing workload studies, but a manager faced with this situation could produce convincing evidence from the workload and shift staffing data to justify her need of more staff.

Workload data is also needed when the client demands for the community midwifery service are taken into consideration.

Section 5.7

Calculating staffing needs for hospital based clinics and parentcraft classes

We have not done, and are not aware of any, workload research on which to base assessment of staffing for clinics. However, the experience of working with maternity services and the more appropriate use of midwives in clinics has enabled us to use the following pragmatic approach to calculating staff needs.

It may come as a relief that we are not going to use any case-mix data.

This is because there is no way of controlling the case-mix as new clients are booked month by month and research into work patterns in general hospital out-patient clinics (Ball, 1986 unpublished) suggested that it is quite valid to use the average length of clinic time as a means of assessing staff needs.

1. Method

To calculate the required numbers of midwives and other staff needed for antenatal clinics, use the following ingredients:

- Number of clinic sessions per week.

- Average length of time taken by each clinic - this can readily be obtained by recording the start of work in preparation for a clinic, the time the first client was seen and the time when the last client left.

- Local practices regarding the deployment of midwives and HCA's or other support staff e.g. history taking, counselling, carrying out antenatal examinations, chaperoning/assisting doctors or midwives, undertaking routine tests, escorting clients to other departments.

For example, a clinic is held every Monday afternoon and is scheduled to start at two o'clock. There are three rooms, two of which are staffed by doctors, the other by a midwife. All of these have the help of a health care assistant.

In addition, there is another midwife who co-ordinates the work of the clinic, ensures clients are booked for scans and escorted to the department etc. A second midwife obtains initial history from new clients and provides advice and counselling primarily for the clients seen by the medical staff.

Two more HCA's carry out routine tests, escort clients to scan department, care for older children, etc as needed.

The normal pattern is as follows. The three midwives and the HCA's begin to prepare for the clinic at half past one; the doctors arrive just before two o'clock. Depending on the number of clients, and their needs, the clinic usually finishes between half past four and five o'clock.

Records kept for three months indicate that the average length of time for the clinic is 3.25 hours, and that the first client was usually seen by five past two.

The staff needed on this pattern is therefore:

- 3.25 hours per clinic x 3 midwives   = 9.75 midwife hours per clinic
- 3.25 hours per clinic x 5 HCA's   = 16.25 HCA hours per clinic.

There is no need to add any allowance for variance, but five per cent is added for management, staff meetings etc.

For this one clinic therefore the following are needed:

- Midwives   =   9.75 + 5 per cent = 10.24 midwife hours per week
- HCA's   =   16.25 + 5 per cent = 17.06 HCA hours per week.

This exercise is undertaken for all the clinics held each week, for example:

Clinic one described above is one of four clinics run every week based on the same methods the staff time needed for the others are as follows:

Clinic 2   =   4 midwives x 4 hours
          =   16 + 5 per cent
          =   *16.8* midwife hours

Clinic 3   =   3 midwives x 2.75 hours
          =   8.25 + 5 per cent
          =   *8.66* midwife hours

Clinic 4   =   4 midwives x 3.65 hours
          =   14.6 + 5 per cent
          =   *15.33* midwife hours

Clinic 1   =   3 midwives x 3.25 hours
          =   9.75 + 5 per cent
          =   *10.24* midwife hours

Weekly midwife hours needed = *51.03*

Allowing for bank holidays the clinics run for 50 weeks per annum
$$= \quad 51.03 \times 50$$
$$= \quad 2551.5 \text{ midwife hours per annum}$$

add 17.3% holiday, sickness etc
$$= 2551.5 \times 1.173$$
$$= 2992.91$$

divide by 52 weeks to obtain weekly hours needed
$$= 57.56$$

Total: 57.56 /37.5 = **1.53 (1.6) w.t.e. midwives to run clinics**.

2. Health care assistants

The number of HCA hours per clinic is as follows:

- Clinic 1 = 16.25 + 5 per cent = 17.06 HCA hours p/wk

- Clinic 2 = 5 HCAs x 4 hours = 20 + 5 per cent = 21.00 HCA hours

- Clinic 3 = 3 HCAs x 2.75 hours = 8.25 + 5 per cent = 8.66 HCA hours

- Clinic 4 = 5 HCAs x 3.65 hours = 18.25 + 5 per cent = 19.16 HCA hours

- Weekly HCA hours needed = 65.88 per week
  x 50 weeks = 3294 hours
  + 17.3 per cent holiday, sickness etc; = 3863.86 hours per annum

- *divide* by 52 weeks to obtain weekly hours needed = 74.31

- 74.31/37.5 **= 1.98 (2.0) w.t.e. HCAs**

3. Flexible working

In many hospitals the clinics are staffed by team midwives who come down from the wards to staff 'their' clinic. This amount of midwife time can be added to that needed for ward areas, providing it is clearly identified. Therefore there may be no need to assess w.t.e for individual clinics to allow for this.

Adding this staff to ward establishment may be of help to small units such as Lakeside to offset the increase above workload needs.

Allowing for change

Using this simple method enables easy adjustment of figures to allow for changes in the deployment of staff. For example, if clinic one became a totally midwife run clinic, then two extra midwives are needed per clinic. As midwives are less likely than doctors to be called away to other areas, the clinics may run for a shorter time e.g.

- Clinic 1
  5 midwives x 3 hours + 5 per cent = 15.75 midwife hours per week
  x 50 weeks = 787.5 hours per annum /52 = 15.14 midwife hours per week
  + 17.3 per cent holidays etc = 17.76 hours/37.5
  = 0.47 w.t.e.

Parentcraft classes/client visits

A similar approach can be taken to assessing staff needed for parentcraft classes, making allowances for the number of classes held per year, and the number of sessions per class or course.

Therefore, if there are 12 courses per year, which run as two classes each week and each course had eight sessions per course:

Two midwives share the running of the courses, both attend the first and last sessions plus another which includes a visit around the hospital, these sessions take up three hours each time.

The midwives then share the other sessions with only one of them attending. These sessions usually last for two hours.

- Midwife time per course
  3 sessions x 2 midwives x 3 hours   = 18 hours
  5 sessions x 1 midwife x 2 hours   = 12.5 hours
  Total per course   = 30.5 midwife hours + *5 per cent*
       = 32.03 hours

- 12 courses per year x 32.03   = 384.3 midwife hours/52
      =   7.39 midwife hours per week
-         + 17.3 per cent   =   8.67 hours/37.5
      =   **0.23 w.t.e midwives**

Section 5.8

Summary: Completing the hospital staffing profile

In the last two units we have seen how:

1.   the case-mix data produced by *Birthrate* helps with the planning of services by:

     a)   forming a basis for planning the number of beds needed by local workload patterns

     b)   provides a means of assessing staff needed on the wards.

2.   Other information about length of postnatal stay and consensus about midwife hours per category day added to the case-mix data:

     •   provides a basis for assessing staff needs
     •   helps with appraisal of different options for managers
     •   demonstrates the impact which different allowances for holidays and sick leave and/or different care policies can have on staffing requirements
     •   illustrates the special needs of small units.

3.   Finally a simple method for assessing staff needed for antenatal clinics and parentcraft classes has been demonstrated.

Producing a staffing profile for hospital services

As we have worked through the last three units, the Birthrate data obtained for each woman passing through the delivery suite has produced a basis for calculating the number of midwives needed to meet required standards of care for intrapartum and postnatal care in hospital.

To this has been added further methods for estimating staff needed for antenatal care, clinics and parentcraft and the number of midwives and health care assisstants required to staff a unit adequately over 24 hours.

To illustrate this, we have put together in the table overleaf the staffing needs for the different departments of Cathedral City which have been produced in the previous units. You may find it helpful to check back just to make sure that you understand how we arrived at these figures.

Staffing needs for Cathedral City hospital services

HOSPITAL SERVICES	MIDWIVES	HCA'S
Intrapartum Care	28	10.94
Ward Based Care	33	17.52
Antenatal Clinics*	0.7	2.00
Totals	61.7	30.46

* antenatal clinics: we have used the example worked out earlier in this unit.

Comment

In the examples given, I have rounded up or down the percentages of staff to whole or at the most one third of a whole time equivalents in all cases where the calculation is based upon workload data. This is because it is not practical to plan staffing in fragments, and because we have to allow for fluctuations in workload, such as midwives needing to work beyond their shift time when the workload is high, some crisis has just occurred or they need to take longer handing over the ward at the shift end.

However, there is not the same need when staff are calculated by shift as in the case of health care assistants or where more staff are allocated by shift then are needed by workload as in the case of smaller units (JAB).

We have not yet addressed any of the issues raised by the implementation of Cumberlege because, as has been shown, there is a need to make a number of decisions about local situations before further decisions can be made about the most feasible and efficient way to develop caseload based work in any particular service. We will address these issues in Unit Six which follows.

Well done!!

If you've managed so far - keep up the good work.
If you're feeling a little daunted - carry on its downhill from here!! (MW).

UNIT SIX

Assessing Staffing Needs for Community Services and Working through Implications of Developing Caseload Based Practice

In this unit we will be using Birthrate and other information to assess staffing needs in the community, whether traditional or caseload based and consider the impact which a number of different care patterns may have on staffing numbers.

Section 6.1: Reviews some of the concepts and definitions of community based midwifery care.

Section 6.2: Looks at the dilemmas raised by the transition to caseload based work, and the strengths and weaknesses of the strategies adopted.

Section 6.3: Explains the principles and staffing formulae used to assess staffing needs for caseload based and traditional care including home deliveries and cross border referrals.

Section 6.4: Demonstrates the calculations for Cathedral City based on the current pattern of traditional care plus some home deliveries and cross-border referrals.

Section 6.5: Works out the staffing implications needs for introducing caseload based care and discusses the implication of four different options for caseload based work.

Section 6.6: Will discuss the need for monitoring the outcomes of the decisions made and controlling workloads.

Section 6.7: Explains how to assess the contribution of caseload midwife time to the staffing needs of the delivery suite, and how this can help in ensuring sufficient core staff for intrapartum care.

Section 6.1

Revisiting the definitions for community midwifery and Cumberlege developments

It might be helpful to begin this section by defining some of the terms used to describe community based midwifery. A number of different terms are being used in this period of change as units make their responses to the Winterton and Cumberlege reports. These have spearheaded the change in care patterns with midwives providing increased continuity of care by working as the lead professional in the care of low risk women, and as the named midwife for high risk women cared for by consultant obstetricians.

Until the advent of these changes a community midwife worked primarily in the client's home and in community based services. The effect of the current changes mean that some midwives now work in the community and in the hospital, taking responsibility as the lead professional. To distinguish between these two types of working therefore we have defined *traditional community care* as that which is mainly restricted to providing antenatal and postnatal care to a woman, but does not involve intrapartum care except where a woman has been booked for a home or domino delivery.

Caseload based midwifery care, developed as a result of the Winterton and Cumberlege reports, means that a midwife provides all aspects of that care; antenatal, intrapartum and postnatal care, including both hospital and home based births. Caseload based midwives may act as the *lead professional* which is a term given by the Cumberlege report to describe the professional (midwife, GP or obstetrician) who takes the primary responsibility for the oversight and care of a woman throughout pregnancy, labour and postnatal care.

Another concept is that of the *named midwife* described in the Patient's Charter, whereby each woman should have a named midwife whose responsibility is to ensure that the client receives the necessary care and who acts as her main contact with the maternity services. In many cases the named midwife will also be the lead professional, but where an obstetrician or GP is the lead professional, a named midwife is also provided. The named midwife may therefore be a hospital midwife, traditional community midwife, or a caseload based midwife.

Further details of these changes and strategies designed to achieve them can be found in the *Cumberlege Report* (1993), and *Effective Group Practice in Midwifery* (Page, 1995).

These changes have faced midwifery managers with a daunting task; how to decide how many caseload based midwifery teams to set up, what workload is appropriate and how to ensure sufficient 'core' staff remain in hospital to ensure all services are adequately maintained?

Section 6.2

Impact of changing community based care in relation to Cumberlege proposals

One of the major principles of Winterton and Cumberlege was that of 'freeing midwives from wards and rotas' so that they could provide woman centred care in different locations according to need.

In particular, it meant that midwives should accompany their women into hospital in labour and remain with them throughout labour and delivery.

Two strategies seem to have been adopted:

1. caseload working midwives are not included in hospital rotas, but work independently in teams or group practices, working in and outside of hospital as required by their clients

2. caseload work midwives work in teams, caring for their clients wherever needed but members of the team are also allocated daily to the rota of staff for the delivery suite, and in some services, to the ante and postnatal wards.

Strengths and weaknesses

The advantages of the *first strategy* is that midwives can work in a fully flexible way, caring for her clients wherever they need her care. This also brings an advantage to the hospital service because the midwife accompanies her client into hospital thus supplementing the labour ward staff in relation to the workload.

The disadvantage is that midwives take on a lot of on-call, which is disruptive to family life, and there is danger of burnout. Part of the answer is to carefully monitor the annual workload of each team or individual midwife and this will be discussed further at the end of this chapter.

The advantage of the *second strategy* is that it avoids excessive on-call for the midwives, but reduces flexibility and efficiency. Midwives may be deployed on the delivery suite when workload is low, but be unable to switch to other duties, because they are needed on the daily roster of staff.

The major disadvantages of this strategy are that it attaches midwives who are trying to provide caseload based work to a rota or shift pattern, which was seen by Winterton as a major block to providing continuity of care.

Clients are less likely to receive care from their 'named midwife', but from whichever member of the team was allocated to the delivery suite at the time. Although many units endeavour to call in the 'named midwife' this may not be possible. This system, therefore, reduces the opportunities for fulfilling the Cumberlege report target of at least 75 per cent of women knowing the person who cares for them in labour.

This system is more likely to create the situation described by Wraight et al (1993) where team midwives feel that they are 'pulled in' from the community based work to staff the hospital services, and where this was not well controlled, it was seen as one of the causes of the breakdown of team midwifery. Such problems are more likely to occur where staffing numbers are short in relation to workload demands.

For these reasons the workload assessment methods recommended take the first strategy as the preferred model.

Other dilemmas

Setting up caseload based work means releasing midwives from hospital rotas or traditional community work. Whether or not managers can afford to do this will depend upon their current establishment. *Therefore, a crucial part of planning is to first assess total staffing needs for a service, and then to examine the feasibility and consequent cost of setting up these systems.*

Factors to be considered include:

- maximum possible flexibility of staff

- ensuring safe staffing levels in the hospital, especially in intrapartum care

- restricting 'fixed' allocation of midwife time in community services in order to free midwives to plan their work in accordance with caseload needs

- preventing overload of community based staff by careful workload control

- combining caseload based working with the 'traditional' community midwife work patterns within a particular service

- providing ante and postnatal care for clients whose maternity care is led by consultants, GP's etc.

Another issue for some services is the need to provide care for cross-border referrals. These are clients who live within the catchment area of a midwifery service but who give birth in another hospital which is either outside the catchment area, or may be a private hospital, and are then transferred back for postnatal care. In some areas these cases produce a heavy extra workload on community based services.

Birthrate has proved an invaluable asset in helping managers to tackle these issues in relation to workforce planning and deployment, because it:

- enables the manager to assess the workload and staff needs of the hospital, thereby indicating core staffing needs.

- the case-mix data more accurately defines low and high risk women, and the outcome category is a firm guide to the patterns of postnatal care which will be required when the woman leaves hospital.

- it also provides a means of assessing the contribution (in terms of w.t.e.) which are made to the staffing needs of a delivery suite by caseload midwives caring for their clients during labour and delivery.

Other reports and recommendations which have influenced methods

Reports which discussed and recommended ways of providing woman focused care by midwifery teams or group practices, assisted in defining the framework for caseload care (Ball et al, 1992, 1995; Page, 1995; Flint, 1991, 1995), and provided the formula which is used to define the required midwife hours per case (Ball et al, 1992). This also helped in defining the midwife hours per case for traditional care.

Recommendations about the size and deployment of teams of midwives and the identification of 'success criteria', shown in the table below, were produced by the report 'Mapping Team Midwifery' (Wraight et al, 1993) and provided the information on the most appropriate team sizes.

Success criteria for team midwifery
- Team consists of no more than six midwives
- Each team has a defined caseload
- Team provides total care for that caseload
- Team works in all areas of client need 50 per cent or more of women are delivered by a midwife known to her (see below)
Source; Box 8.1: Wraight et al., 1993

The Cumberlege Report recommended that,

'At least 75 per cent of women should know the person who cares for them during delivery'.

Section 6.3

Principles of planning for traditional and caseload based care

1. Using the case-mix data to define workload especially in terms of low and high risk cases, intrapartum care, length of postnatal stay in hospital.

2. i) Planning initially based on caseload team/group practice numbers of six midwives each caring for 35 -38 cases per midwife per annum (Ball et al, 1992, 1995; Wraight et al, 1993; Flint, 1995; Page 1995)

   ii) Planned numbers will be affected by geography factors and case-mix. The results of the second year of the One to One Midwifery Service (Page et al, 1996) indicated that where workload is well controlled, and distances between the clients homes and the hospital are limited, midwives can successfully handle 40 cases per annum.

3. Applying the formula for midwife hours per case - either caseload work which includes hospital births and/or home deliveries or traditional midwifery care.

4. Adding midwife hours needed for ante and postnatal care for cross-border referrals.

5. Allowances for administration concerned with the running of the group/team and meetings with managers or for undertaking audit, etc.

6. Travel allowances; these may vary from one area to another.

7. Whole-time equivalents are based on total midwife hours per annum = 1612.5 hours per annum (as shown earlier, p.90, Unit 5, Section 2).

Producing a formula for estimating midwife hours per client

The following formula was first produced by a team of expert midwives who met together on a number of occasions in 1991 in order to debate the feasibility and methods of providing within the National Health Service, the type of midwifery care which it was thought would be recommended by the Winterton Committee. The result was published (Ball et al, 1992) to coincide with the publication of the Winterton Report.

Since then the formula has been updated. Antenatal hours have been reduced in line with the Cumberlege recommendations, and increased hours are given for the postnatal care of complicated or high risk cases (defined by *Birthrate* as Categories IV and V), to allow for extended visiting both at home and in hospital.

In many units, caseload based midwives care for all women within a catchment area whether they are high risk or low risk.

---

1. Formula for assessing midwife hours per client for caseload based work (hospital or home delivery)

Antenatal care	*Hours*
Booking visit/ initial planning etc.	1.5
Ultrasound	0.5
Antenatal contacts at 26, 34, 36, 38, 40 weeks	5.0
Parentcraft, hospital visits for client and partner	2.0
Total =	*9.0*

Intrapartum care
(includes labour, delivery and follow-up visit or discharge from hospital within six hours and includes some allowance for a second midwife to attend a home delivery)

Total =	*17*

Postnatal care: includes visits at hospital or home

1. **Low risk**/normal outcomes:
   transferred from hospital on 1st - 3rd day postnatal *and* discharged around 10th to 12th day.
   12 visits as needed   *10* hours

2. **Complicated cases** requiring longer postnatal care in hospital
   transferred from hospital 4-7 days
   discharge around 15-18th postnatal day   *15 hours*

Note: The stated number of days does not refer to daily visits, but the span of days when midwife would attend.

Total hours per case:
Normal/low risk
36 hours per case + 5 per cent admin/management =   *38 hours*

Complicated/high risk
41 hours per case + 5 per cent admin/management =   *43 hours*

Administration allowances

The hours per case given in the two formulae include all the direct and indirect care i.e. paper work, telephone contacts, etc for each client. Study leave is included in the staffing hours per annum.

Administration allowances of five per cent account for team/group meetings and liaison which are additional to contacts related to client care, plus meetings with managers, audit, etc. (five per cent equals two hours per case over and above client related administration).

---

2. Formula for assessing midwife hours for traditional care of clients delivered by hospital staff

Antenatal care (all cases)
Assuming that the midwife is involved in shared antenatal care with GP and hospital, but does not act as lead professional

6.5 hours + 5 per cent administration	=	*7.0 hours per case*

Postnatal care
1. Low risk
Early transfer home; Days 1-3; discharged by midwife around days 10/12 =

8.5 + 5 per cent	=	*9.0 hours per case*

2. High risk/complicated
Home 4-7 days, discharged by midwife around day 13-16 =

7.0 + 5%	=	*7.5 hours per case*

Total hours:
low risk	=	*16.0 hours*
high risk; complicated cases	=	*14.5 hours*

(*Note:* complicated cases need less time because the midwife does not visit in hospital as the caseload based midwife would). Travel allowances also need to be added.

Travel allowances

There seems to be a dearth of information on the amount of midwife time spent travelling around and between clients homes, the hospital, community services etc. Where local data are available via Korner or other audit procedures, then that is the travel allowance which should be added to the midwife hours required.

Where such data are not available the following recommendations may be of help to managers. These have been produced as the result of working with maternity units in large cities, market and industrial towns and in rural areas. Also we have indicated the increase of hours per care of the various percentage allowances as this demonstrates some of the increased costs of community care in different geographical locations.

TRAVEL ALLOWANCES AND WORKING LOCATIONS

In the examples given below, we have shown how much is added to the total time for normal cases by the percentage travel allowance given. For example, 10 per cent of 38 hours equals 3.8 hours. In the case of complicated cases, where the staffing formulae required 43 midwife hours per case, a travel allowance of 10 per cent would add 4.3 hours per case. Therefore, travel allowances will make a higher increase where midwives care for a mixed caseload of normal and complicated cases, or where they cover a wide geographical area.

- Ten per cent: mainly urban; not heavily congested; small radius for clients within ten miles of bases (3.8 hours for each normal case)

- 15 per cent: mainly urban; with some rural, covering a wider radius of up to 15 mile radius of base (5.7 hours for each normal case)

- 17.5 per cent: either heavily congested urban area (e.g. central areas of main cities) or mixed urban and rural area with radius of up to 20 miles from base (6.65 hours for each normal case)

- 20 per cent: mainly rural; longer distance into main unit; radius of 20 - 40 miles for caseload midwives (7.6 hours for each normal case).

Allowances above 20 per cent should be verified by local data and are likely to be needed in rural areas with limited road systems e.g. North of Scotland, Lake District, parts of East Anglia.

Section 6.4

Estimating community staffing needs

Before this can begin, a number of questions need to be addressed, and the answers will depend on the degree to which a service has already changed or plans to change to caseload based working:

1.   How many women need care from the community each year from main hospital, home deliveries, cross border referrals?

2.   What is the pattern of work?

Is workload all caseload based i.e. midwife takes full responsibility for care including the delivery?

Is workload all traditional i.e. midwife provides ante and postnatal care but not responsible for full care/delivery?

Is workload a mixture e.g. mainly caseload, plus extra postnatal care for hospital based cases or mainly traditional plus some domino and/or home deliveries a year?

3.   In either case, what is the case-mix for which the midwives are responsible. i.e. all low and high risk cases in a geographical area or low risk only?

Calculating midwives needed depends on sorting out the different care needs, the way care is organized, calculating the midwife hours for each of these and then adding them together to make a whole.

Let us take Cathedral City again as an example:

The manager already knows how many midwives she needs for the hospital services, (see last section) and from the *Birthrate* case-mix she knows how many cases could be classified as low and high risk.

Now she needs to assess her community staffing needs, and wishes to decide how many caseload teams to set up.

In addition to the hospital births of 3000 per annum, there were 24 home deliveries (16 in city and 8 in rural area) and 210 cross border referrals who received ante and postnatal care from the rural area midwives.

In the current situation, how much is the community workload and what staff are needed?

Cathedral City Hospital
3000 births per annum and annual Birthrate casemix

	I	II	III	IV	V	TOTAL
% casemix	10.8	36.9	19.2	14.2	18.9	100
No. cases p.a.	324	1107	576	426	567	3000
No. days stay in ward	2	2	3	5	7	

From the information shown in the familiar table above, and counting all the Category I-III cases as *low risk/normal* and those in IV and V as *high risk/complicated*:

- there are 2007 cases (67 per cent) who will be transferred home within one to three days *(Categories I-III)*

- 993 who will come home after the fifth postnatal day *(Categories IV and V)*.

In addition care is needed for 24 home deliveries and 210 cross-border referrals.

Based on existing traditional care patterns the number of midwives can be calculated thus:

1. Hospital births
    2007 normal cases x 16 hours per case   = 32112 midwife hours
    993 complicated cases x 14.5 hours per case   = 14398.5 hours

    Total midwife hours including administration   = 46510.5

    Add a travel allowance of 15 per cent   = 46510.5 x 1.15
    = Midwife hours per annum   = 53487.1
    = 53487.1/1612.5   = *33.2 w.t.e. midwives*

2. *Add 24 home deliveries* at 38 hours per case = 912 hours
    + 15% =1048.8 midwife hours/1612.5   = *0.65 w.t.e.*

3. *Add 210 cross border cases*

Records do not exist about how many of these cases were low or high risk, therefore the managers bases her calculations on a similar case-mix as her own:

- 70 per cent of 210 = 147 low risk x 16 hours   = 2352 midwife hours
- 30 per cent of 210 = 63 high risk x 14.5 hours   = 913.5 midwife hours
- Total   = 3265.5 midwife hours + 15 per cent
         = *3755.33/1612.5*   = *2.33 w.t.e.*

Therefore total number of midwives needed for traditional care =

- hospital births   33.20 w.t.e.
- home deliveries   0.65 w.t.e
- cross-border   2.33 w.t.e.

    Total =   **36.18 w.t.e.**

(Current staffing = 48 w.t.e midwives)

Section 6.5

Making plans to introduce caseload based care
Option one
The manager decides to start *caseload* work with four group practices of six midwives per team, and to develop them in the City area close to the hospital *thereby reducing the travel allowance for these cases to ten per cent.*

Each team will care for *220* women per annum and will care for both *low* and *high* risk categories, plus *sixteen home deliveries* spread among the teams according to client need (This figure is based on last year's patterns in the City area).

The remaining clients including eight home deliveries and the cross border referrals will be cared for by traditional midwives as at present.

Planning the workloads
Planning is based on the *Birthrate* data which shows that 67 per cent of cases are in Categories I - III and 33 per cent in IV and V.

Therefore, the manager plans on the caseload midwives caring for 70 per cent low risk and 30 per cent high risk women.

Based on 880 cases = 616 low risk and 264 high risk women

	LOW RISK	HIGH RISK	TOTAL
Caseload midwives	616	264	880
Traditional midwives	1391	729	2120
TOTALS	2007	993	3000

Assessing staffing needs for caseload work
- 616 x 38 hours   = 23408 midwife hours
- 264 x 43 hours   = 11352 midwife hours
- Total   = *34760 midwife hours*

A travel allowance of ten per cent is added because these midwives are working in a smaller radius:

$$= 34760 \times 1.1$$
$$= 38236 \text{ midwife hours per annum}$$

- *38236/1612.5* $= 23.71 \text{ w.t.e midwives}$

Add 16 home deliveries at 38 hours each $= 608 + 10 \text{ per cent}$
$$= 668.8/1612.5 \quad = 0.41 \text{ w.t.e.}$$

Total planned workload for caseload work needs
$$23.71 + .41 \quad\quad\quad\quad = \textbf{24.12 w.t.e.} \text{ midwives}$$

Given the lee-way already built in on hours per case for normal deliveries it is likely that this workload could be managed by **24 w.t.e. midwives** (this means that each midwife cared for 37-38 women per annum).

Assessing staffing needs for traditional care

As shown above, these midwives will care for 1391 low risk and 729 high risk women:

- 1391 low risk x 16 hours $= 22256.0 \text{ midwife hours}$
- 729 high risk x 14.5 hours $= 10570.5 \text{ midwife hours}$

Total hours = *32826.5* midwife hours per annum + 15 per cent travel. As these cases will be spread around the city outskirts and the surrounding rural area:

- 32826.5 x 1.15 $= 37750.5 / 1612.5$
$$= 23.41 \text{ w.t.e. midwives}$$

Add eight home deliveries as before:

- 8 x 38 hours = 304 hours + 15% = 349.6 / 1612.5
$$= 0.22 \text{ w.t.e.}$$

Add 210 cross border cases $= 2.33 \text{ w.t.e.}$

Total for traditional care:

- $= 23.41 + 0.22 + 2.33$
- **= 25.96 (26) w.t.e. midwives**

Summary of option one

Total midwives for 3000 hospital births:

* 2120 cases (traditional care)
* 880 cases (caseload work)
* 24 home births and 210 cross border referrals plus caseload work in the City area = 50.08 (50) w.t.e. (24 w.t.e. caseload 26 w.t.e. traditional) which is an increase of 2.08 w.t.e. over the current staffing and 13.9 w.t.e. more than needed for traditional care alone.

Dilemmas and options

The manager now has a problem. Changing to caseload based working in one area means an increase of two whole-time equivalents, and she is not likely to gain the extra funds for this unless she can make a very good case. She therefore needs to consider other factors which might offset costs, or demonstrate improved quality of care. These now need to be built into her planning and option appraisal before she seeks the funding required.

Factors to be addressed

INPUT TO DELIVERY SUITE BY CASELOAD MIDWIVES

One of the benefits of caseload working is that the midwife comes in with her client once labour is established, thus supplementing the staff needed by workload. In units caring for a higher number of births per annum than Cathedral City this can be a considerable input. The manager therefore assesses how much midwife time will be contributed to the delivery suite staff by the caseload based midwives.

Note that full details of how to assess this input from the case-mix data will be explained more fully at the end of this section.

For our example, the manager considers that as the midwives are working close to the hospital and are not carrying a heavier than recommended workload (Ball et al, 1992; Flint; 1995) then they should be able to care for at least 75 per cent of their clients throughout labour and delivery. These should include both low and high risk cases.

On the pattern shown in *Option one* therefore, if caseload = 880:

* 75 per cent of 880 = 660 women
* 660 women = 22 per cent of all births (660/3000x100=22 per cent).

Therefore the caseload midwives are expected to deliver 22 per cent of all hospital based births.

From the calculations made for Cathedral City and shown earlier in Unit 3 (p.46), the manager knows that she needs **28 w.t.e. midwives** for intrapartum care.

If the *caseload midwives* care for 22 per cent of all births then that work is equal to **6.16 w.t.e midwives.**

Therefore caseload working could reduce the staff needed for delivery suite by six whole time equivalents which would offset the costs of two extra midwives in the community (see Section 7, p.40).

However, before she can go further the manager needs to check that reducing the delivery suite staffing to **22 w.t.e.** will ensure sufficient numbers of midwives on each shift.

ENSURING ENOUGH CORE STAFF FOR DELIVERY SUITE

In considering this issue, the manager concludes that the minimum core staff per shift is *four midwives*, and from the examples shown earlier in Unit 5 (p.101) we know that four midwives per shift day and night = *23 w.t.e.*

The manager may decide that she needs to retain extra midwives for the days when elective caesarean sections take place, and so she would maintain the core staffing at *24 w.t.e.*

Therefore the input from caseload based midwives would allow a reduction of *4 w.t.e.* in the delivery suite staffing figures.

OTHER POTENTIAL REDUCTIONS IN HOSPITAL WORKLOAD

Although not of the same significance as reducing staffing needs in the delivery suite, implementing caseload based working should result in a decrease in *Category X* admissions, and in the number of women attending antenatal clinics which should produce a further albeit a small reduction in staff on the wards and in the clinics.

Summary of option one

	Low Risk	High Risk	TOTAL	w.t.e. Midwives
Caseload midwives	616	264	880	23.71
Traditional midwives	1391	729	2120	23.41
TOTAL				47.12
Add 0.41 w.t.e. and 0.22 w.t.e. for home deliveries				0.63
Add cross border referrals				2.33
TOTAL				50.08

Staffing would be planned at *50 w.t.e.*

Although the first results indicated that creating four caseload teams meant an increase of 2 *w.t.e.* above current staffing in the community of *48 w.t.e.* we can see that adopting this option provides an opportunity for reducing the hospital based staff by *four w.t.e.* which means that Option one could be achieved and produce a reduction of *two w.t.e.* in the *total staff needed for Cathedral City*.

Other options

The manager can show that the increase in the community services are off-set by their contribution to delivery suite staffing and organization. She may also want to consider other options which might reduce the costs of introducing caseload based working.

She could do this by calculating the staffing needs if:

a)   caseload midwives cared for low-risk cases only *or*
b)   she had three caseload teams rather than four

(Remember: Option one = four caseload teams caring for high and low risk women).

Option two: caseload deal with low risk only

The care of complicated cases needs more midwife time, thus allocating only low risk women to caseload care would reduce staffing needs, but would impact on quality of care as many would argue that it is even more important to provide continuity of care to high risk women. Nevertheless, where financial restrictions are high, it may be the only way to *initiate* caseload based patterns of care.

In our example therefore; the midwife hours needed would be:

*   880 low risk hospital births and 16 home deliveries
        = 896 x 38 hours
        = 34048 hours + 10 per cent
        = 37452.8/1612.5
        = **23.23 w.t.e.**

This is not a large reduction compared to the *24.14* needed for high and low risk women, and would reduce the number in one team below that recommended by Wraight et al (1993).

This is because the only change is a reduction from 43 hours for high risk women to 38 hours per case for low risk.

Option two: traditional midwives

The traditional caseload would also change. There would be an increase of 264 high risk women previously allocated to caseload care but a corresponding decrease of 264 low risk women.

This is shown below:

Allocation of cases to different midwife groups

	Low Risk	High Risk	TOTAL
Caseload midwives	880	-	880
Traditional midwives	1127	993	2120
TOTALS	2007	993	3000

Traditional midwife staffing needs:

- Low risk workload = 1127 cases x 16 hours = 18032 hours
- High risk workload = 993 x 14.5 hours = 14398.5 hours
- Total = 32430.5 hours

- + 15% travel = 32430.58 x 1.15
  = 37295.08 hours
- Divide by 1612.5 = *23.13 w.t.e.*

Summary for option two

- Caseload midwives: low risk only + 18 home deliveries = 23.23
- Traditional midwives: 23.13 w.t.e + 8 home deliveries = 0.22 w.t.e
  + cross-border referrals = 2.33
- Total = *25.68 w.t.e.*

Total for Option two = **48.91 w.t.e. (49 w.t.e.)**

Staffing would be planned at *49 w.t.e.* which is a reduction of *1 w.t.e.* from Option one. This does not seem a great advantage when one considers that high risk women do not have the opportunity to receive caseload based care.

Delivery suite contribution

The contribution to the delivery suite would change because the caseload midwives are now caring for a percentage of low risk women only, and Categories I-III need less midwife time than do those in Categories IV and V.

If the caseload midwives again deliver 75 per cent of their booked cases equalling 660 low risk women, their contribution to the delivery suite staff would amount to *33 per cent* of all low risk women.

This is worked out below but this time the method is a little more complicated.

Firstly, we need to calculate how many midwives are needed in the delivery suite to care for all the low risk women (=2007) then we can assess how much of this work will be provided by the caseload midwives.

(The full details of how to assess the input of caseload midwives to delivery suite workload is shown at the end of this section.)

We turn back again to the intrapartum data.

Cathedral City Hospital
Birthrate data on 3000 births per annum

	BIRTHRATE CATEGORIES					
	I	II	III	IV	V	TOTAL
% casemix	10.8	36.9	19.2	14.2	18.9	100
No. cases p.a.	324	1107	576	426	567	3000
Mean daily no.	0.89	3.03	1.58	1.17	1.55	
W/load ratios	1.0	1.34	2.14	2.6	4.2	
W/load index	0.89	4.06	3.38	3.03	6.52	

Staff needed for low risk cases:
If we take the total work-load index for low risk cases only (I-III) then this is:

- 0.89 + 4.06 + 3.38   = 8.33

Using the same number of midwife hours per Category I as before, the staff needed for this work load is:

- 8.33 x 5.9 midwife hours = 49.15 x 7 days   = 344.03
  + 15 per cent   = 395.63 hours + 5%   = 415.42 hours
  add 17.3% leave etc   = 487.28/37.5
                                              = *12.99 w.t.e.midwives*

(The staff needed for high risk women would be 14.9 w.t.e.)

Therefore if caseload midwives deliver 33 per cent of all low risk women, they will contribute 4.29 w.t.e. midwives' worth of time (12.99/100 = 0.13 x 33 = 4.29).

Therefore the manager can plan on *reducing* the delivery suite staff by **4 w.t.e.** as in Option one.

(*Remember* in Option one the caseload input was *6 w.t.e.* but the manager needed *24 w.t.e.* if she was to ensure four midwives per shift as a minimum core staff, plus one other w.t.e. for peaks of workload).

COMPARISON OF OPTIONS
Option one: 50 w.t.e. (50.08)
Option two: 49 w.t.e. (49.32)

Option three caseload: three teams only

Another option might be to reduce the number of teams to three, and calculate the workload based on:

a) low risk women only
b) mix of high and low risk as in *Option one*.

If there are three teams of six midwives caring for 660 births and 16 home deliveries then the w.t.e. needed are:

a) *Low risk only*
660 x 38 = 25080 +10 per cent   = 27588 midwife hours
27588/1612.5   = 17.11 w.t.e. midwives
+ 16 home deliveries   = 0.41 w.t.e

                                       = *17.52 w.t.e. in total*

b) *Low and high risk*
70 per cent of 660 = 462 x 38   = 17556 hours
30 per cent of 660 = 198 x 43 hours   = 8514 hours
Total   = 26070 hours

+ 10 per cent   = 28677 hours/1612.5   = 17.78 w.t.e. midwives
+ 16 home deliveries   = 0.41 w.t.e
                                       = **18.19 w.t.e. in total**

Traditional midwives

There would be an increase in the workload of the traditional midwives as they would now have 200 more women to care for.

The distribution for *Option three* is shown below:

Allocation of cases to different midwife groups

		Low Risk	High Risk	TOTAL
a)	Caseload midwives	660	-	660
	Traditional midwives	1347	993	2340
	TOTALS	2007	993	3000
b)	Caseload midwives	462	198	880
	Traditional midwives	1545	795	2340
	TOTAL	2007	993	3000

Calculating traditional midwives on option three a.

*   1347 low risk x 16 hours = 21552 hours + 993 high risk
                              = 993 x 14.5
                              = 14398.5

Total hours   = 35950.5 + 15 per cent travel
               = 41343.08/1612.5
               = 25.64 w.t.e. midwives

Add 0.22 (home deliveries)
and 2.33 (cross border) = **28.19 w.t.e**.

Calculating traditional midwives on option three b.

*   1545 low risk x 16 hours = 24729 hours + 795 high risk
                              = 795 x 14.5
                              = 11527.5

Total hours   = 36247.5 + 15 per cent travel
               = 41684.63/1612.5
               = *25.85 w.t.e. midwives*

Add 0.22 (home deliveries)
and 2.33 (cross border) = *28.4 w.t.e*.

Summary of option three

	Caseload midwives	Traditional midwives	TOTAL
Option 3a	17.52	8.19	45.71
Option 3b	18.0	28.4	46.6

INPUT TO THE DELIVERY SUITE

Based on the caseload midwives delivering 75 per cent of their booked cases as before, then the contribution to the delivery suite for:

Option 3a (low risk cases only) would be *2 w.t.e.*

Option 3b (low and high risk cases) would be *3 w.t.e.*

Making decisions

Now the manager must decide which option to go for. The various results are compiled in the following table:

SUMMARY OF OPTIONS FOR CATHEDRAL CITY

Current establishment for community services: *48 w.t.e*

Using *Birthrate* data on 3000 births per annum + 24 home deliveries and 210 cross-border referrals the staff needed for different patterns of midwifery care are:

Based on traditional care only: *36.18 w.t.e.*

Choosing preferred option

This must be done by the local managers debating the costs and benefits of the various options.

The comparison of staffing numbers, allowing for the contribution to delivery suite staffing:

- Option 1:   46.00 w.t.e.
- Option 2:   45.32 w.t.e.
- Option 3a: 43.71 w.t.e.
- Option 3b: 44.60 w.t.e.

Although the preferred option might be Option 1, thus implementing four caseload teams providing care for high and low risk women, this might not be financially viable *in the first year.*

Although *Option 3a* is the least costly, it does not provide the best quality option for high risk women. Nor does Option 2.

Therefore if the cost of *Option 1* is too high, the next best would be Option 3b which would enable a model of caseload working to be tested, and provide the basis for further development.

There may be other benefits in choosing Option 3b or Option 1. There is evidence (Page et al, 1995, see section 3) that providing caseload teams who care for high and low risk women significantly reduces the *length* of postnatal stay in hospital. However, this benefit would not be apparent until some time after implementing caseload based working.

In the example shown in the second version of ward staffing, the reduction in ward staff amounted to *6.13 w.t.e.*

The full implications of these options are shown in the total summary of staffing for Cathedral City, shown opposite, and which sets the staffing figures in the context of defined client workload and care policies. Some of the figures shown opposite were discussed earlier in Units 3 and 5.

BASED ON INTRODUCING CASELOAD BASED CARE:

Summary of options	Caseload	Traditional	Total	Delivery Suite
Option One				
4 teams:				- 4
high + low risk	23.41	23.41		
home births	0.41	0.22		
cross-border	-	2.33		
TOTAL	24.12 (24)	25.96 (26)	50.08	- 4
	(in 'real' terms = 50 - 4 = 46 w.t.e.)			
Option Two				
4 teams:				- 4
low risk only	23.23	23.13		
home births	0.41	0.22		
cross-border	-	2.33		
TOTAL	23.64	25.68	49.32	- 4
	(in 'real' terms = 49.32 - 4 = 45.32 w.t.e.)			
Option Three				
a) 3 teams:				- 2
low risk only	17.11	25.64		
home births	0.41	0.22		
cross-border	-	2.33		
TOTAL	17.52	28.19	45.71	- 2
	(in 'real' terms = 45.71- 2 = 43.71 w.t.e.)			
b) 3 teams:				- 3
high + low risk	17.78	25.85*		
home births	0.41	0.22		
cross-border	-	2.33		
TOTAL	18.19	28.40	46.59	- 2
	(in 'real' terms = 46.6- 2 = 44.6 w.t.e.)			

* the higher number of traditional midwives is because they have an increase in low risk cases who need more traditional time, than the high risk women who stay in hospital longer.

Summary of total staffing needs for Cathedral City

The staff shown below are based upon:

1. Demand:
   3000 hospital births, 24 home deliveries, 210 cross- border referrals.

2. Care policies: processes and outcomes
   Birthrate outcomes and case-mix which reflect population needs and intrapartum care policies.

   Alternative lengths of stay for ante and postnatal care.

3. Organization and deployment of staff:
   Number of midwives and HCA's for hospital service based on the above workloads, policies and care patterns.

   Different options for community work.

   Clearly defined allowances for travel and holiday, sickness and study leave.

The results are as follows:

Staffing needs for Cathedral City Maternity services

HOSPITAL SERVICES	MIDWIVES	HCAs
Intrapartum care		
a) current patterns of care from hospital midwives	28	10.94
b) minus contribution from caseload teams:		
Core staff: Options 1 and 2 - 4	24	10.94
Option 3a - 2	26	10.94
Option 3b - 3	25	10.94
Ward based staff		
On current length of stay	33	17.52
Antenatal clinics	0.7	2.00
TOTALS		
a) current patterns	61.7	30.46
b) Options 1 and 2 in community	57.7	30.46
c) Option 3a) in community	59.7	30.46
d) Option 3b) in community	58.7	30.46

Note: The total staffing numbers shown above include time for co-ordinating care and day to day team/ward management. However, they do not include any clinical specialist or senior management staff.

Antenatal clinics and parentcraft

This was not done specifically for Cathedral City, but we have used the example of four clinics shown in Part 3 which is typical of this type of unit.

It can be seen that in the case of Cathedral City Maternity Services implementing caseload based teams has the potential to reduce the hospital staffing needs by a range of 2-4 w.t.e.

However this needs to be set against the staff needed for the various options in the community.

Total staffing needs for Cathedral City maternity services based on four options for caseload based care

In the list below we have put the *full* staffing because we have already made allowances above for the contribution to delivery suite staff.

Total Staff needed:	Community	Hospital	Total w.t.e.	
Option 1	50.00	61.70	111.70	(112)
Option 2	49.32	57.70	106.82	(107)
Option 3a	45.71	59.70	105.41	(105)
Option 3b	46.60	58.70	105.30	(105)

Final decisions

Putting the total figures together, it can be seen, that if it is not possible to fund Option 1, then Option 3b provides the most cost and quality efficient alternative. It is perhaps surprising to note how much difference is made by changing the mix of clients for caseload based midwives.

In the case of Option 3 although 3b needs 0.89 w.t.e. more in the community than Option 3a, it provides one full w.t.e. midwife more to the delivery suite staffing.

How feasible will it be to develop caseload based care?

It can be seen in the staffing figures for Cathedral City that the degree to which caseload based care can be developed will depend upon:

- differences between current staffing establishment and that needed for development

- amount of hospital staffing which can be off-set against caseload based development

- the amount of distance to be covered by caseload and traditional midwives and its impact upon travel allowances.

In the case of Cathedral City these are not insuperable, and experience suggests that many services caring for 3000 women a year or more will have enough lee-way in the current staffing establishment to make the change. However where services are being expected to make arbitrary cuts in staffing to meet budget reductions there may be considerable difficulty in moving forward.

The same is true of *small units* who have already been highlighted in terms of their increased needs of staff to meet 24 hour demand for hospital services. Many of these units provide care in widespread rural areas, and this adds to their problems in developing caseload based work, not least because the addition of the higher travel allowances mean that the number of midwives per number of clients is increased.

For example, in Cathedral City four teams of six midwives were caring for 880 women per annum with a travel allowance of ten per cent.

- If we use the same mix of 70 per cent low risk and 30 per cent high risk then we need the same midwife hours per annum = 34760 but this time,

- 17.5 per cent travel is added = 40773.5 midwife hours/1612.5 = 25.3 w.t.e. midwives rather than 23.71 shown earlier (before adding 16 home deliveries).

This means that small units face a number of problems:

a) increased travel costs per client

b) the need to provide extra staff in hospital means that there is less opportunity for off-setting these costs by the contribution made by caseload midwives to hospital based care.

This discussion will be taken up again in the last chapter.

This section will end by first returning to the need to monitor the clinical and personnel outcomes of management decisions and of regularly reviewing actual workload patterns.

This will be followed by the details of how to assess the caseload based midwives input to delivery suite staffing needs.

Section 6.6

Monitoring the outcomes of decisions made

Once a decision has been made, it is advisable for the manager to set up a system of monitoring:

- the actual numbers of home and hospital births

- the percentage cared for during labour by caseload midwives

- the number and case-mix of women cared for by the two types of community midwives, and their length of stay in hospital for postnatal care

- similar data should be collected for any cross border referrals.

It is also important to continue to collect *Birthrate* data as an ongoing measure of demand and care outcomes.

This will enable the manager to:

- assess the effectiveness of the reorganization to practice by comparing the percentages of women booked for caseload care who were cared for during labour by a) their named midwife, b) another member of the same team or group, or c) by hospital core midwives who were not previously known to the client.

- assess the degree to which the projected or estimated number and case-mix of births matched the actual demand and assess the impact of any significant difference.

- investigate whether any change in demand was due to increase or decrease in volume or was due to changes in care strategies.

and as a result

- make more specific plans for the following year.

The next chapter will deal further with adjusting staffing needs according to planned or unplanned changes.

Monitoring workloads

It would be naive to suppose that, having produced workforce plans and care strategies that they will continue as intended without regular review and where needed, adjustment.

Wraight et al (1993) pointed out the danger of uncontrolled or vague workloads being managed by team midwives. Experience in helping maternity services has demonstrated that there can be considerable problems if workload is not controlled.

This has arisen in two ways:

1. enthusiastic or parochial caseload midwives who have booked far more women per annum than was planned

2. managers who have expected caseload based midwives to take on 'extra' hospital booked women because of staff shortages or because the total workload has not been properly worked out.

One way of identifying an effect of excessive workload is to monitor the percentage of booked cases who are delivered or attended in labour by their booked midwife.

Where this is considerably lower than the expected target, this should be urgently investigated. In one situation a particular team of caseload based midwives pioneering the new service as one of four teams each covering a postal area, booked a total of 278 women over the year, when their planned target was 210. Perhaps it was not surprising to find that 45 per cent of these women were not cared for in labour by their named midwife or one of the other team members, but by a hospital midwife who was not known to the client, thus defeating the object of caseload work.

The reason given was that this team of midwives did not want to pass on the 'extra' cases to their colleagues in the other caseload based teams, nor to their hospital colleagues. But in effect that was happening during intrapartum care!

In another hospital, where caseload based midwives worked on a rota system and were deployed daily in either the delivery suite or the wards as well as in the community, the percentage of women delivered by caseload teams was stated to be 65 per cent. However, when individual case notes were examined, only 22 per cent of women had been cared for during labour by their booked midwife, 43 per cent by another member of the team of six midwives, and the remainder by hospital midwives previously unknown to them. This situation came to light as the result of complaints from women who had been led to expect individual care from their *lead professional* and who were extremely disappointed.

In an different maternity service, the manager said that the caseload based midwives were 'occasionally' asked to provide traditional type care to clients who lived within the catchment area of the team. When monitored by reviewing care records it was found that a team who booked 225 women for full care had been asked to take a total of 98 'extra' cases during the year. This *occasional* extra work needed 1.12 w.t.e. midwives!

These examples of failure of the caseload based system were due to excessive workload, or to a pattern of deploying midwives which worked against the flexibility needed for achieving the pattern of continuity upon which caseload based work is founded.

Another problem which has come to light in hospital services is the lack of or insufficient 'core' staff for delivery suite and the wards. Where proper provision has not been made, midwives have been called away from the care of their clients in order to staff peaks or crises in workload.

Perhaps it is not surprising that such problems have occurred in the initial development of Cumberlege type services, but it is crucial that they are not allowed to continue. If they do the service will eventually flounder, not because of lack of ability or commitment but because of bad management and organization.

This unit will close with an explanation of the method for assessing the input which caseload based midwives make to delivery suite staffing.

Section 6.7

Working out caseload midwives contribution to delivery suite staffing

When midwives 'come in' to attend and/or deliver their booked cases, they contribute to delivery suite staffing.

In many situations this means that delivery suite can be reduced by the contribution made by caseload working midwives. However it is crucial to ensure that there is sufficient 'core' staff always available.

Principles

The principles are explained via another example given below:

1. Intrapartum workload and staffing needed:

    *   Determine how many births per annum and the Birthrate case-mix e.g.= *4000 births*
    *   Work out staffing via mean hours per case, workload indices and the staffing formula
    *   Staff needed for this workload e.g. = 38 w.t.e. midwives.

2. How many caseload teams e.g. eight teams of six midwives?
    How many cases will they book for care per team e.g. 210 per team x 8 = 1680?
    What is the target?
    How many do you expect they will deliver or attend in labour e.g. 75 per cent?

    Therefore in this example caseload based midwives are expected to deliver or attend in labour 1260 women during the year (1680 x .75 = 1260).

3. What is the caseload mix? Do they book both low and high risk?
    if Yes, proceed as shown opposite
    if No, use method shown later.

1.   Method when mix is low and high risk cases

This is the easiest to work out. We can assume that caseload midwives cases match general case-mix. Therefore we can calculate what percentage of total workload they will be responsible for:

- 1260 women = 31.5 per cent of total workload on delivery suite
  (1260/4000 x 100 = 31.5 per cent)

Therefore caseload based midwives will provide 31.5 per cent of total care needed.
- Total midwives for delivery suite= 38 w.t.e.
- 31.5 per cent of 38 = 11.97 (12) w.t.e.
- (38/100 x 31.5)   = 11.97)

In this example caseload midwives contribute 12 w.t.e. worth of midwife time to delivery suite needs.

Staff needed therefore =   Core staff = 26 w.t.e.
                            Caseload contribution = 12 w.t.e.
                            Total = 38 w.t.e.

Check if there are enough core staff to provide a minimum of 4/5 midwives per shift.

- 4 midwives per shift   = 23 w.t.e
- 5 midwives per shift   = 28.75 w.t.e.

Therefore deducting the caseload contribution from total staffing will still provide adequate cover from the core staff round the 24 hours.

2.   Method for low risk only caseload

This is a little more complicated to work out as the midwives will be providing care to a particular section of the workload which usually has a lower input of midwife time. Of course some of the booked cases may become high risk but the planning is based on low risk only.

a).   How many will midwives deliver?
       Midwives book and attend low risk cases only, and deliver or attend in labour 85 per cent of all booked cases = 1428 women (1680 x .85 = 1428)

b).   What is total low risk workload?

Add up the numbers of cases in each of the Categories I, II and III.

In this example:

- Cat I = 524 cases
- Cat II = 720 cases *and*
- Cat III = 936 cases

Total   = 2180 low risk cases

Therefore if caseload midwives care for 1428 low risk cases, then they will care for 66 per cent of all low risk cases: (1428/2180 x 100).

3.   How many staff are needed for total low risk case-mix ?

	CAT. I	CAT. II	CAT. III
% Mix	13.1	18.0	23.4
No. per annum	524	720	936 = 2180 births
Daily mean =	1.4	2.0	2.6
Workload ratios	1	1.4	2.4
Workload =	1.4	2.8	6.2
Workload index =	10.4		

- Midwife hours per category I   = 5.6 hours
  Staffing needed   = 10.4 x 5.6
                                                    = 58.24 hours per day
      58.24 x 7   = 407.68 hours per week
      + 15% variance   = 407.68 x 1.15
                                                    = 468.83 hours
      + 5% management   = 468.83 x 1.05
                                                    = 492.27 hours
      + 17.3% hols etc   = 492.27 x 1.173
                                                    = 577.44 hours / 37.5 hours
                                                    = **15.4 w.t.e. needed for low risk workload**

Caseload midwives care for 66% of these cases = 10.16 w.t.e. 'worth' (15.4 x .64 = 10.16).

Staff required for intrapartum care on delivery suite:

Example One   Mixed *low* and *high* risk caseload

CORE	CASELOAD	TOTAL
26	12	38

Example Two   Low risk caseload only

CORE	CASELOAD	TOTAL
28.14	9.86	38

UNIT SEVEN

Managing Change

In this final unit we will be looking at how to review and reassess staffing needs, in the light of changes in demand upon a service and the effect which local factors have upon staffing needs.

Section 7.1:   Reviewing and reassessing staffing needs.

Section 7.2:   Raise the question of how to reassess staffing needs in the light of planned or anticipated change:

        a)   in the number of births per annum
        b)   in the number and case-mix of births per annum

Section 7.3:   Explores again the impact of case-mix and local factors upon staffing needs and asks whether there is an ideal size for a maternity unit.

Section 7.1

Reviewing and reassessing staffing needs

Introduction

We have now come to the final part of the workforce planning model which was described in Unit 1 and is repeated below.

Assessing the demand
- Clinical indicators of client need, quality targets combine to produce initial staffing options ↓

- Using professional judgement to address quality and geography issues.

↓

Making management decisions
- Reviewing options and making decisions in relation to unit wide priorities, demands, targets and constraints ↓

- Coming to final decision on staffing numbers for a defined period of time in relation to defined care objectives

↓

- Plans made for regular review and reassessment of staffing needs.

Rather like the quality cycle, once decisions have been made, the process of assessing staffing needs begins again. Plans must be put into action which will enable continuing review and reassessment of staffing needs in the light of changes in the demand for service.

One of the main problems facing health service managers is the degree to which they have been forced to manage in a reactive way. Staffing numbers have largely been a matter of historical development, possibly affected by changes in the service, such as an extension of the number of beds, or the appointment of extra consultants. Rarely have they been reviewed in the light of changes in clinical practice for midwives (e.g. introduction of epidural services), or changes in the number of births per annum because of population change, closure of other units or attracting new contracts from other purchasers.

Managers have found themselves caught between their desire to encourage expansion of services and development of midwifery skills, and their fear of not having sufficient resources to meet the challenge.

Although it is not a magic wand, *Birthrate* data can help in making a more pro-active response, by assessing in advance, the effects which such changes may have upon unit workload and the staffing response needed to maintain quality standards. This enables managers to determine the feasibility of coping with the anticipated or proposed change as part of the option appraisal process.

Keeping an eye on Birthrate data

One of the purposes of continuing to collect *Birthrate* data is that it can act as an early signal of unplanned or unexpected change. For example, where a new consultant or obstetric registrar is appointed who has a different care policy from his predecessor.

Any marked or unexpected change in the percentage case-mix over several months should be investigated. It may be due simply to a cluster of high or low risk cases which will even out over time, or it may be due to a change in policy, which will need to be discussed. Another reason for unexpected change in the case-mix is that incorrect data is being produced, usually by new staff who have not been properly instructed in its use or purpose. The monthly audit of data which was discussed in Unit 3 is vital and should be regarded as an integral part of unit information.

Section 7.2

Dealing with planned or anticipated change

As we have seen in the previous sections of the handbook, staffing needs are based upon a defined number of hospital and home births per annum plus any other work such as cross border referrals. Once the staffing numbers have been agreed, the budget is set. Therefore any significant change in the volume of births or case-mix will create change in the number of staff required.

These changes may be expected due to a planned uptake of work, which may be a particular issue in these days of competition among provider units in some densely populated areas, or it may be anticipated based on a change in the local population of women aged 15-44, or it may be unexpected. Sometimes an increase in volume is also accompanied by a change in case-mix.

A change in the number of births and or case-mix needs an assessment of staff requirements. To illustrate this we will look at two examples:

1.   Change in the number of births

Growmore Unit's staffing plan is based on a total of 4000 births per annum which was the average number in previous years. For the last two years, the birth rate was 4250 and 4350 and the local population statistics indicate that this is likely to continue, as the population of women aged 15-44 will remain stable for the next few years.

The manager decides to plan her staffing for the next three years on 4300 births per annum.

2.   Change in both volume and case-mix of births

Allchange Unit serves a large urban district where the decision has been made to close a small maternity unit which is sited on the edge of the town and has cared for a steadily falling number of women for a number of years.

The last two years the number of births has been around 1000 a year. In addition a consultant obstetrician based at the smaller unit is about to retire. The main unit will now provide care for all these women as well as the 3500 they normally care for.

In these examples, the methods will be demonstrated by calculating the staff needed for intrapartum care, but further calculations would need to be made for the wards and community based care.

Calculating staff needs where the number of births change: Growmore Unit

The method is fairly simple. The manager is dealing with a rise in existing volume, and as the same clinical policies will be in operation there is no need to make any adjustments to the case-mix. Therefore, the managers reassesses her staffing based on her existing case-mix which is applied to the new total of births per annum.

Growmore unit is based in a large DGH and has an intensive neonatal care unit as well as a large delivery suite with twin theatres. It serves a mixed urban and rural population.

Current workload and staff needed: intrapartum care

The existing *Birthrate* data shows the following case-mix and staffing needs for current volume of 4000 births per annum.

Growmore Unit	I	II	III	IV	V	TOTAL
% casemix	15.7	19.8	20.5	22.4	21.6	100
Numbers =	628	792	820	896	864	4000
Daily mean =	1.7	2.2	2.25	2.45	2.37	
W/load ratios	1	1.7	2.4	3.4	4.3	
W/load index	1.7	3.74	5.4	8.33	10.2	29.37

- Workload index   = 29.37
- Midwife hours per case   = 5.4
- Midwife hours per day   = 29.37 x 5.4
                                   = 158.6
- Midwife hours per week   = 158.6 x 7
                                   = 1110.19
- +15% variance (x 1.15)   = 1276.71
- +5% management (x 1.05)   = 1340.55 midwife hours/37.5
                                   = 35.75 w.t.e.
- +17.3% (x 1.73) holidays, sickness etc   = 41.93 (42) w.t.e.

Now the manager needs to:

1. Calculate the number of cases per category based on the same case-mix and 4300 births per annum e.g. 15.7% of 4000 = 628
   15.7% of 4300 = 675 (4300/100 x 15.7)

2. Work out the new daily mean number of cases and the workload indices. The workload ratios per category and the mean hours per Category I remain the same.

The results are:

Growmore Unit	BIRTHRATE CATEGORIES					
	I	II	III	IV	V	TOTAL
% casemix	15.7	19.8	20.5	22.4	21.6	100
Numbers =	675	851	882	963	929	4300
Daily mean =	1.85	2.33	2.42	2.64	2.55	
W/load ratios	1	1.7	2.4	3.4	4.3	
W/load index	1.85	3.96	5.81	8.98	10.97	31.57

- Workload index   = 31.57
- Midwife hours per case   = 5.4
- Midwife hours per day   = 31.57 x 5.4
                                      = 170.48

- Midwife hours per week   = 170.48 x 7
                                      = 1193.36

- +15% variance (x 1.15)   = 1372.39
- +5% management (x 1.05)   = 1441.01 midwife hours/ 37.5
                                      = 38.43 w.t.e.

- +17.3% (x 1.173) holidays, sickness, etc   = 45.07 w.t.e. (45 w.t.e.)

Adding 300 births per annum on this case-mix means an increase of 3 w.t.e. midwives for intrapartum care.

Note: this unit has 44 per cent of its cases in Categories IV and V.

Assessing staffing needs for the rest of the service

Further calculations should be made by working through all the other areas of care: postnatal and antenatal care on the wards; antenatal clinics; caseload and traditional community care.

Calculating staff needs where the number of births change and the case-mix changes: Allchange Unit

This time there is a change in the volume of births because of the closure of the smaller unit and a possible change in the case-mix.

The smaller unit had one 'resident' obstetrician who has now retired and two others who were based in the main unit provided a part-time service and emergency cover. The retirement of the obstetrician has coincided with the closure of the unit. A new consultant has been appointed at the main unit to accommodate the extra cases. No *Birthrate* data is available from the smaller unit.

In this example the manager could simply add 1000 cases to her existing volume of births and the existing case-mix and calculate the staff needed on that basis. However, most of the women cared for at the smaller unit fell into the *low risk* category: elective caesarean sections were not carried out; there was no epidural service and any antenatal problems were transferred to the main unit as early as possible.

The small unit records show that of 1000 women delivered at the unit in 1995. 135 (14 per cent) required emergency caesarean section:

* 135 (14 per cent)   required emergency caesarean section
* 285 (29 per cent)   needed assisted delivery
* 22 (2.2 per cent)   babies were transferred to the main unit for neonatal care.

The manager decides to define the emergency caesareans as Category V, the sick neonates and their mothers as Category IV and the assisted deliveries as Category III.

She also anticipates that a fair percentage of women will take advantage of the epidural service at the main unit and estimates that at least 15 per cent will do so.

Her estimate of the Birthrate outcomes for the women who would normally have been delivered in the small unit is as follows:

* 135 caesarean   (Cat V cases)
* 285 assisted deliveries   (Cat III)
* 22 sick neonates   (Cat IV)

* Total = 442 women (some of these would have had an epidural).

This leaves 558 more.

If ten per cent of the remaining 558 women elect for epidural = 56 (which means that Cat III now = 341 cases), this leaves 502 women to be distributed between Categories I and II.

These are shown in the table below:

Birthrate Categories for the new 1000 cases p.a:

	I	II	III	IV	V	TOTAL
Numbers	200	302	341	22	135	1000

Birthrate data from the main hospital:

	BIRTHRATE CATEGORIES					
	I	II	III	IV	V	TOTAL
% Casemix	16.4	22.5	23.4	19.7	18.0	100
Numbers =	574	788	819	689	630	3500
W/l ratios	1	1.65	2.1	3.3	4.0	

Midwife hours per Category I = 5.35 hours.

If you would like to work out the mean daily numbers and the workload indices and staffing please do so.

The answer should be 32.56 w.t.e. midwives for intrapartum care.

Now we will work out the staff needed for the new number and case-mix of clients:

Birthrate Categories for the new 1000 cases p.a:

	I	II	III	IV	V	TOTAL
Numbers	200	302	341	22	135	1000

The manager adds the numbers per category from the 1000 new cases to the numbers per category for the existing 3500 cases and works out the new case-mix. The results are:

	BIRTHRATE CATEGORIES					
	I	II	III	IV	V	TOTAL
Numbers =	774	1090	1160	711	765	4500
% Casemix	17.0	24.0	26.0	16.0	17.0	100
W/load ratios =	1	1.65	2.1	3.3	4.0	

Midwife hours per category I = 5.35 hours.

If you would like to work out the daily mean and the staffing numbers based on the above, please do so.

The answer should be 40.41 w.t.e. for intrapartum care.

So in this example, increasing the workload by 1000 cases means that an increase of 7.85 w.t.e. are needed in the delivery suite.

The reason for the difference lies primarily in the case-mixes of the two units.

In Growmore Unit 44 per cent of cases were in Categories IV and V and it had slightly higher workload ratios.

The existing data for Allchange Unit showed that 37.7 per cent of cases were in Categories IV and V. Adding the primarily low risk cases from the smaller unit resulted in a case-mix where only 33 per cent were in the Categories IV and V. This reduction is significant because the higher the category the greater the number of midwife hours needed. This influence will continue throughout the rest of the staffing needs for the wards and community care services.

Section 7.3

Effect of case-mix and local factors upon total staffing

Pitfalls in comparing midwife/client ratios

The examples of data given in this handbook clearly demonstrate the impact which clinical policies and facilities can have upon the workload. The larger units with specialist services care for a larger percentage of high risk clients from their own catchment area as well as those clients who are transferred for specialist maternal or neonatal care from other units. Conversely, smaller units will have a proportionately lower percentage of high category clients.

The examples we have used in the manual, Cathedral City and Lakeside, are real examples of these smaller units, and this can be seen in their case-mixes. Therefore their staffing needs will be proportionately less per number of clients than the larger specialist units.

In the examples just shown, Growmore and Allchange, the data is more typical of the larger units. There is no real place for suggestions of special virtue for smaller units, but each unit should review its case-mix in the light of what it considers to be 'good outcomes' given the clientele it caters for and the services it provides.

For this reason, one must be wary of making simplistic comparisons between units, such as clients per midwife assessed by dividing the total number of midwives in a service by the number of births. In at least one Regional Health Authority a list has been drawn up which gives ratios of deliveries by number of midwives in 21 different hospitals. While it is not suggested that this becomes a basis for assessing appropriate staffing, one can foresee the temptation for purchasers to quote these figures as a basis for costs per case.

Is there an ideal size for a maternity service?

Maternity Units in England and Wales seems to lie in three different size bands:

- 3000-4500 births per annum
- 4500-6000 or more births per annum
- *and* smaller units which vary from less than 1000 births, 1000-2000 or 2000-3000.

Units which care for 3000 births or more per annum will probably have sufficient flexibility in their staff numbers to develop some degree of caseload based working. The larger units will have a much greater freedom to do so. These are some of the issues which need to be taken into consideration when planning for Cumberlege developments. Not all units will be as able to meet the targets as others.

A further obstacle to caseload working in smaller units is the larger distances and travel costs involved, and where minimum staff levels must be maintained to provide 24 hours cover in the hospital, flexibility in staff deployment is reduced. As a result caseload midwives may find themselves carrying a large amount of on-call duties, and this is not easy to maintain for long periods of time.

But slightly larger units which cater for 2500-3000 births a year may also fall into this category if their case-mix has a high proportion of low risk women, which is more likely in small units!

What is the solution?

In some areas, the answer has been to close the smaller units and merge their cases with those already being cared for by a larger unit within the same area. But many of the smaller units serve widespread rural areas, where there are large distances to cover before reaching a larger unit, areas where road communications are not good, either because of winding roads or congested in the summer period. In many of these areas the client population is expanded by tourists.

In such situations closing the unit would significantly reduce the availability of care across a wide area of population.

The answer seems to be that it will be necessary for health service purchasers and general managers to accept that these units serve a clear need, cannot be readily replaced and therefore will need to have a higher midwife/client ratio because of their special staffing needs.

Issues of how to evaluate the efficacy and relevance of the organization of midwifery care will become a major issue, and sound methods must be used and further developed. A forthcoming book will provide valuable insight into these issues (Garcia and Campbell, 1996 in press).

Final Comments

In this manual we have sought to provide managers with a clinically based framework for assessing workforce needs.

Previous sections of the manual have focused upon different aspects of maternity care and patterns of midwifery organization, and raised issues of decision making in each area.

We have shown that there is no set answer to the question 'how many midwives?' because a number of local issues and decisions impinge upon the final answer.

We have shown however, how the components and processes of workforce planning and decision making shown earlier in Part 1 can be applied to midwifery care. The main processes of that model were described as:

---

1. Assessing the demand – clinical indicators of client need, quality targets combine to produce initial staffing options.
   ↓
2. Professional judgement is used to address specific issues to assess quality and geography issues and their impact on decision making. Appraising the strengths and weaknesses of different options.
   ↓
3. Making management decisions – reviewing options and making decisions in relation to unit wide priorities, demands, targets and constraints.
   ↓
4. Making final decision on staffing numbers for a defined period of time in relation to defined care objectives.
   ↓
5. Plan to set up methods for review and reassessment.

As we have progressed through the various sections we hope that this process has become a little clearer. In the model of Cathedral City we have built up a total staffing profile for a medium sized unit based upon a number of care options.

We have also touched on the staffing needs of a small unit and one large unit (Majorport) in order to demonstrate the differences which local situations make.

What we have not done

Although we have touched on skill mix in terms of midwives and health care assistants needed in different areas of care, and have planned on the basis of health care assistants providing family type care to clients and acting as assistants to midwives, we have not raised the issue of grade mix among midwives. Decisions about grade mix will depend upon local situations and organization of services. Managers must make those decisions for themselves.

Neither have we addressed maternity leave because this is not an issue which affects all staff each year, and therefore cannot be added as a set allowance to the staffing formulae. Managers must make their own assessment of the likely impact of maternity leave on their services.

Another issue is that of specialist clinical and management staff above that needed for day to day co-ordination of services. Again these are matters for local decisions, but it is important that they are not overlooked.

The issue of staffing for neonatal services has not been addressed because we have not had experience in developing methods for these services. However, we consider that the clinical categories of need produced by the Report of the British Association of Perinatal Medicine and the Neonatal Nurses Association (1992) would provide a firm basis for developing a method for assessing nursing hours needed per client category, but would need to be expanded to include care of parents as well as infants.

The need for sound management and monitoring of workload, team management and client outcomes has been discussed in the context of different aspects of care and in the light of the pitfalls awaiting team/caseload midwifery so well set out by Wraight et al (1993).

As the book has progressed we have shown the use of various staffing formulae. There will be found listed separately in the appendices so that readers can readily use them for their own workload/workforce calculation.

All the calculations shown in the *Birthrate* system can be done with a simple calculator, although the use of computer spreadsheets will make the task easier.

In many units computer based record systems have been adapted to produce the *Birthrate* scores and categories. The use of computer analysis should also be accompanied by the random independent audit of *Birthrate* record described in Unit 3, to ensure that correct data are being recorded in the system. Monthly checks of the resulting data are also recommended so as to identify any unexpected changes in the case-mix of midwife hours per case. Such events usually indicate that incorrect data has been input.

Computer companies are also reminded that the *Birthrate* systems described in this handbook remain under copyright. Although they may be freely used within the National Health Service, full reference and acknowledgement of the author should be shown on all documents, and permission sought for any commercial exploitation.

We hope that we have not offended any reader by spelling out things which were already well understood. Our objective was to provide existing and future managers with a well reasoned and illustrated framework for understanding the demands made by their client workload and the options which they may need to address as they face the task of balancing the demands for cost-effectiveness, client satisfaction and quality of care, safety, the maintenance of staff morale and the expansion of midwifery skills and responsibilities.

As Handy (1985) so pithily put it,

> 'is the manager a masochist or is there something in the job of linch-pin which imposes this kind of life on him (her)? A bit of both seems to be the answer!'

It is to these linch-pins, the managers of midwifery, that this book is dedicated.

Glossary

Definitions and glossary of terms used in workload measurement and staffing issues, and in midwifery services

These lists are provided to help clarify terms used in the text, especially to readers who are either not familiar with workforce planning issues or with commonly used midwifery terms. In discussion with midwives and other managers we found that there were often difficulties in defining some of the new patterns of midwifery care, and so we have attempted to do so.

Overseas readers may find these lists helpful in understanding the various patterns of midwifery organization current in the United Kingdom.

Midwifery terms used in the manual

The list of midwifery terms is drawn from a number of publications which include:

- House of Commons (1992). *Report of the Health Committee on Maternity Services* Chair: Winterton. Vol.1, London: HMSO.

- Department of Health (1993). *Changing Childbirth Report of the Expert Maternity Group Part 1.* Chair: Cumberlege. London: HMSO.

- Page, L. (1995). *Effective Group Practice in Midwifery.* Oxford: Blackwell Science

annual hours per midwife:
> a means of deciding staffing needs by assessing total hours per annum provided by one whole-time equivalent midwife, after deductions for holidays and a small allowance for sickness and study leave.

antenatal care:
> the skilled oversight and support provided during pregnancy with the objective of ensuring as far as possible the health and well-being of the woman and her baby. Its pattern should ensure that 'the woman and her partner feel supported and fully informed throughout the pregnancy and are prepared for the birth and care of their baby' (Cumberlege, 1993).

apgar scores:

a scoring system devised by an anaesthetist, Virginia Apgar (1953), which is used to assess the condition of the infant at birth

a score of 0, 1 or 2 is given to five factors: heart rate, respiration, muscle tone, reflex response and colour

a normal infant in good condition will score 7-10. A lesser score means the infant requires some resuscitation.

birth plans:

a written plan completed after discussion between the woman and her midwife/ GP/obstetrician which details the woman's wishes for the management of her labour and delivery.

caseload based midwifery care:

developed as a result of the Winterton and Cumberlege reports, in which the midwife acts as lead professional in managing the care of the woman and provides all aspects of that care - antenatal, intrapartum and postnatal care. Includes both hospital and home based births.

community midwife:

a midwife who works primarily in the woman's home and in community based services.

continuity of care:

ensuring the organization of maternity care enables a woman to develop a 'relationship built on trust with those looking after her and ensure that one of them is with her at crucial times such as the birth' (Cumberlege).

cross-border referrals:

women who live within the catchment area of a midwifery service but who give birth in another hospital outside the catchment area, and are transferred back for postnatal care. Clients who have received private care are also included in these referrals. In some areas they produce a heavy extra workload on community based services.

Cumberlege:

the colloquial term used for the reforms of maternity care spearheaded by the Winterton Report and detailed in the objectives and targets set by the Report of the Expert Group on Maternity Care chaired by Baroness Cumberlege.

domino deliveries:

> this term is given to deliveries in which the community midwife accompanies her client into hospital, provides the necessary intrapartum care, and the woman returns home within a few hours of the birth (The term was coined from 'Domiciliary midwife in and out').

home deliveries:

> where a woman gives birth at home cared for by her community midwife and wherever possible her general practitioner.

intrapartum care:

> providing the skills, knowledge and empathy needed to care for and support a woman throughout labour and delivery, providing the human and technical resources required and taking such action as is needed to ensure, as far as is possible, the health and well-being of the woman and her baby. After the birth this care includes the encouragement of close and uninterrupted contact between the mother, her partner and their baby and completing all necessary medical and legal documentation.

lead professional:

> a term arising from Winterton and Cumberlege Reports meant to specify the professional (midwife, obstetrician or GP) who takes the primary responsibility for the oversight and care of a woman throughout pregnancy, labour and postnatal care.

midwife-led units:

> hospital or GP unit services in which the clinical care is managed entirely by midwives, who refer clients to consultant oversight if necessary.

midwife teams:

> a system of organizing midwives into teams which care for a particular group of women. They may be made up of caseload based, community or hospital midwives.

named midwife:

> concept described in the Patient's Charter whereby each woman should have a named midwife whose responsibility is to provide her with the necessary care. In many cases the named midwife will also be the lead professional, but where an obstetrician is the lead professional a named midwife is also provided.

parentcraft classes:
> special classes held as part of antenatal care.

postnatal care:
> providing the skills, knowledge and support required to promote the physical and emotional well-being of the woman and her baby, and to prepare the woman and her partner for the continuing care of their child/children.

shared care:
> the term given to the sharing of the total care of a woman between her GP, community and hospital midwives and obstetrician.

staffing the rota:
> describes midwives working on a shift by shift basis, either in hospital or community in which her allocation of time and duties are pre-fixed.

staffing the women:
> a term first found in the Winterton report which distinguishes between the type of midwifery practice which allows midwives the flexibility to work with her clients wherever and whenever her skills are needed, rather than working on a rota basis within a particular ward or department.

traditional community care:
> care which is mainly restricted to providing antenatal and postnatal care to a woman, but does not involve intrapartum care except as a home or domino delivery.

Terms used in workload and workplace planning
Many of those used in workload/workforce planning systems are drawn from:

Hurst, K. (1993). *Nursing Workforce Planning.* Harlow: Longman.

This book provided the first comprehensive analysis and review of all nursing workforce planning systems and special thanks are due to Keith Hurst for his permission to use his excellent glossary.

Other sources include:

Ball, J.A., Goldstone, L.A., Collier, M. (1984). *Criteria for Care - the Manual of the North West Nurse Staffing Levels.* Project Newcastle-upon-Tyne Polytechnic Products Ltd, Newcastle-upon-Tyne Polytechnic.

Ball, J.A., Hurst, K., Booth, M.R., Franklin, R. (1989). *But Who Will Make the Beds? A Research-based Strategy for Ward nursing Skills and Resources for the 1990s.* Leeds: Nuffield Institute for Health University of Leeds. 71-75 Clarendon Road Leeds LS2 9PL.

Ball, J.A., Hurst, K. (1990). 'Signs for the times' *Health Service Journal* 29th April, Vol. 100, No. 5198, pp.632-534.

activity analysis:
analysing the patterns of nursing activities within a defined area, recorded at pre-set time intervals, to produce a profile of distribution of nursing time and skills to different aspects of care.

Most valid method is by non-participant observation. Best done over 24 hours and eight consecutive days.

acuity:
in workload/workforce literature, means the average dependency per patient for a ward/speciality. Can be used as a nursing demand indicator and to distinguish changes in workload over time or difference between different wards.

associated work:
generally used for non-nursing work such as serving meals, routine or general clerical work and manning telephones.

bed occupancy:
the number of occupied beds in a ward expressed as the percentage of the whole.

clinical indicators:
> describes criteria which indicates the patient's degree of illness/need for medical and nursing care and to which is given a comparative score so that a total score indicates the degree of need.

direct care:
> hands on care provided by nurses to a patient.

establishment:
> a term given to the agreed numbers of nursing staff required for a ward, department, total hospital or community service, which includes holidays, sickness and other allowances.

indirect care:
> individual but remote patient care e.g. writing a report, telephoning for a doctor, arranging for discharge, etc.

nursing workload:
> indicators of the amount of nursing time required to provide appropriate care to a group of patients.

patient dependency:
> a classification system which allocates patients to one of several categories arranged in a hierarchical manner that denotes increasing degrees of need for nursing care.

ratios:
> a means of showing the relative size of a one number compared to another e.g. 12 = 1.2 times the number 10, 30 is nearly twice the size of 18, its ratio is 1:1.66.

staff in-post:
> the staff assessed as required for the day to day running of a ward or department, which does not include any allowances for holidays, sickness or other allowances.

whole time equivalent (w.t.e.):
> one way of expressing the staff required by a service and is equal to the total hours worked by a full-time member of staff. Currently 37.5 hours per week.

> A part-time member working 23 hours per week = 0.6 w.t.e. (can sometimes be expressed as full-time equivalent f.t.e.)

workload index:
> a number which expresses the total workload of a ward or department, which is produced by multiplying the number of patients in each dependency group by the workload ratios for that group and adding them together.

workload ratios:
> indicate the comparative workload for patients in different dependency groups.

References

Apgar, V. (1953). 'A proposal for a new method of evaluation of the newborn infant'. *Current Research in Anaesthesiology and Analgesics.* 40, p.340.

Audit Commission (1992). *Caring Systems: A Handbook for Managers of Nursing and Project Managers.* London: HMSO.

Auld, M. (1976). *How Many Nurses? A Method of Estimating the Requisite Nursing Establishment for a Hospital.* London: Royal College of Nursing.

Ball, J.A., Goldstone, L.A., Collier, M. (1984). *Criteria for Care - the Manual of the North West Nurse Staffing Levels.* Project Newcastle-upon-Tyne Polytechnic Products Ltd, Newcastle-upon-Tyne Polytechnic.

Ball, J.A., Oreschnik, R.W. (1986a). 'Criteria for care' *Senior Nurse.* Vol. 5, No. 4, October pp.26-29.

Ball, J.A., Oreschnik, R.W. (1986b). 'Balanced formula' *Senior Nurse.* Vol. 5, No. 5, Nov/Dec pp.30-32.

Ball, J.A. (1987). 'A quality environment' *Senior Nurse.* Vol. 6, No. 1, Jan pp.23-24.

Ball, J.A. (1986). *Why Are We Waiting?* A Study of North Lincolnshire Health Authority Out-Patient Service Internal Report NLHA, Lincoln.

Ball, J.A. (1988). 'Dependency levels in the delivery suite' In: *Proceedings of the Research and the Midwife Conference* pp.2-24.

Ball, J.A. (1989). *Birthrate: A Method of Outcome Review and Manpower Planning in the Delivery Suite* (Unpublished). Leeds: Nuffield Institute for Health Services.

Ball, J.A., Hurst, K., Booth, M.R., Franklin, R. (1989). *But Who Will Make the Beds? A Research-Based Strategy for Ward Nursing Skills and Resources for the 1990s.* Leeds: Nuffield Institute for Health University of Leeds. 71-75 Clarendon Road Leeds LS2 9PL

Ball, J.A., Hurst, K. (1990). 'Signs for the times' *Health Service Journal* Vol. 100, No. 5198, pp.632-34.

Ball, J.A. (1992). *Birthrate: Using Clinical Indicators to assess Case-mix, Workload Outcomes and Staffing Needs in Intrapartum Care and for Predicting Postnatal Bed Needs.* Leeds: Nuffield Institute for Health University of Leeds.

Ball, J.A., Garvey, M., Jackson-Baker, A., Flint C., Page L. (1992). *Who's Left Holding the Baby? An Organisational Framework for Making the Most of Midwifery Services.* Leeds: Nuffield Institute for Health University of Leeds.

Ball, J.A. (1993). 'Workload measurement in midwifery' In: Alexander, J., Levy, V., Roch, S. (Eds). *Midwifery Practice; A Research-based Approach.* Basingstoke: Macmillan.

Ball, J.A., Garvey, M., Jackson-Baker, A., Flint, C., Page, L. (1995). 'Who is left holding the baby? Meeting the Challenge of the Winterton Report' In: Page, L. (Ed). *Effective Group Practice in Midwifery* Oxford: Blackwell Science Ltd.

Barr, A. (1967). *Measurement of Nursing Care.* Oxford: Oxford Regional Hospital Board.

Barr, A., Moores, B. (1972). *Nursing Dependency as a Basis for Staff Deployment.* Oxford: Oxford Regional Hospital Board.

Barr, A. (1984). 'Hospital nursing establishments and costs' *Hospital and Health Service Review.* January pp 31-37. Oxford: Oxford Regional Hospital Board.

Bell, A., Storey, C. (1984). 'Assessing workload by a nursing study' *Nursing Times* Vol. 80, No. 34 pp.57-59.

British Paediatric Association and Royal College of Obstetricians and Gynaecologists (1977). *Recommendations for the Improvement of Infant Care during the Perinatal Period in the UK: A Discussion Document.* London: BPA/RCOG.

British Paediatric Association and Royal College of Obstetricians and Gynaecologists (1982). *Midwife and Nurse Staffing and Training for Special Care and the Intensive Care of the Newborn: A Consultation Document.* London: BPA/RCOG.

British Perinatal Society and the Neonatal Nurses Association (1992). 'Report of the working Group of the British Perinatal Society and the Neonatal Nurses Association on categories of babies requiring neonatal care'. *Archives of Disease in Childhood* Vol. 67 pp.868-869.

Department of Health and Social Security (1980). *The Second Report from the Social Services Committee on Perinatal and Neonatal Mortality.* Chair: Short. London: HMSO.

Department of Health (1993). *Changing Childbirth Report of the Expert Maternity Group Part 1;* Chair Cumberlege. London: HMSO.

Flint C. (1995). 'Being and becoming the named midwife' In: Page, L. (Ed). *Effective Group Practice in Midwifery.* Oxford: Blackwell Science.

Garcia, J., Campbell, R. (1986). *The Organization of Midwifery Care: A Guide to Evaluation.* Hale: Hochland and Hochland Limited (in Press).

Goldstone, L.A., Ball, J.A., Collier, M. (1983). *Monitor: An Index of the Quality of Nursing Care in Acute Medical and Surgical Wards* Project Newcastle-upon-Tyne Polytechnic Products Ltd Newcastle-upon-Tyne Polytechnic.

Handy, C.B. (1985) *Understanding Organizations* (3rd Edition) Middlesex, England: Penguin Books.

House of Commons (1992). *Report of the Health Committee on Maternity Services.* Chair; Winterton. Vol.1, London: HMSO.

Knaus, W.A., Zimmerman, J.E., Wagner, D.P., Draper, E.A., Lawrence, D.E. (1981). 'APACHE - Acute Physiology and Chronic Health Evaluation; a physiologically based classification system' *Critical Care Medicine* Vol. 9, pp.591-597.

Knaus, W.A., Zimmerman, J.E., Wagner, D.P., Draper E.A., Lawrence D.E. (1981). 'Evaluating outcome from intensive care: a preliminary multihospital comparison'. *Critical Care Medicine* Vol. 10, pp.491-496.

Maclean, G., Bowden, H.I. (1988). 'Developing a midwifery workload management system: a preliminary report' *Midwifery* Vol. 5, pp.172-181.

Maternity Services Advisory Committee (1985). *Maternity Care in Action; Part II Intrapartum Care* London: HMSO.

Morgan, C.J. (1986). 'Severity scoring in intensive care'. *British Medical Journal* Vol. 292 p.1546 June.

NHS Management Executive (1993). *A Study of Midwife and GP-led Maternity Units NHS Management Executive* London: Department of Health.

Page, L. (1995). *Effective Group Practice in Midwifery.* Oxford: Blackwell Science.

Page, L., Lathlean, J., Campbell, M., Vail, A., Piercy J., Wilkins, R. (1995). *Progress Report; One to One Midwifery Practice Internal Paper,* Centre for Midwifery Practice, Hammersmith Hospitals NHS Trust and Thames Valley University.

Page, L. (1996). Personal communication.

Rhys-Hearn, C. (1974). 'Evaluation of patient's nursing needs: prediction of staffing; Occasional Papers 1-4' *Nursing Times* Vol. 70, pp.69-84.

Scottish Home and Health Department. (1969). *Nursing Workload as a Basis for Staffing Report by the Work Study Department of the North Eastern Regional Hospital Board.* Scotland.

Senior, O. (1979). *Dependency and Establishments: A Study of General Hospital Wards.* London: RCN.

Telford, W.A. (1983). *Determining Nursing Establishments; the Telford Consultative Approach* Sutton Coldfield: North Birmingham Health Authority.

Trent Health (1991). *Report of the Trent Midwifery Manpower Planning Project.* Ed: Tierney, M. Trent RHA.

Washbrook, M. (1993) *Report on Length of Stay by BIRTHRATE Category.* Personal Communication

Washbrook, M. (1995). *Data on Length of Stay by BIRTHRATE Category from Two Maternity Hospitals.* Personal Communication.

Wraight, A., Ball, J., Seccombe, I., Stock J. (1993). *Mapping Team Midwifery: A Report to the Department of Health Institute of Manpower Studies Report Series 242.* Brighton: Institute of Manpower Studies.

APPENDIX ONE

Birthrate Score Sheet

BIRTHRATE SCORE SHEET

Mother's details		Date of delivery		199
		Length of time in delivery suite		hours

Section A	**GESTATION / LABOUR / INTERVENTIONS**		
Gestation	37 weeks or more	1	
	More than 34 weeks, less than 37	2	
	Less than 34 weeks	3	
Length of labour	8 Hours or less	1	
	More than 8 hours	2	
As required	I.V. infusion (*not blood transfusion*)	2	
	Epidural in situ	3	
	Elective general/spinal anaesthetic	3	
	Continuous fetal monitoring	3	
(see note on multiple birth scores)	Twins*	2	
	Triplets, quadruplets, etc*	5	
	Medical problems needing consultant oversight *e.g. diabetes, heart or chest conditions*	5	
	Subtotal SECTION A		

Section B	**DELIVERY**		
	Normal delivery	1	
	Forceps / breech, etc	2	
	Elective Caesarean section	3	
	Emergency Caesarean section	5	
** Must be scored for caesarean section	**Perineum intact	1	
	Vaginal/perineal tear/episiotomy	2	
	Extended episiotomy/3rd degree tear	3	
	Subtotal SECTION B		

Section C	**INFANT(S)**		
Apgar assessed at 5 minutes	Apgar score 8+	1	
	Apgar score between 5 and 7	2	
	Apgar score less than 5	3	
Multiple births : score each baby	Birth weight 2.5 kg or more	1	
	Birth weight 1.5kg - 2.5kg	2	
	Birth weight less than 1.5kg	3	
As required	Congenital abnormality	3	
	Infant is stillborn / dies immediately after birth	5	
	Subtotal SECTION C		

Section D	**OTHER INTENSIVE CARE**		
	I.V. infusion **started or maintained** post-delivery	2	
	Blood transfusion at any stage of labour	5	
	Emergency general/spinal anaesthetic	5	
	Intensive care not accounted for by any other factor	5	
	Subtotal SECTION D		

TOTAL SCORES AND INDICATE CATEGORY AS SHOWN BELOW			
Score 6 =	Category I	Score 14 - 18 =	Category IV
Score 7 - 9 =	Category II	Score 19+ =	Category V
Score 10 - 13 =	Category III		
		Other Categories	X A R

HAVE YOU CALCULATED LENGTH OF TIME IN DELIVERY SUITE ....?

* J A Ball Nuffield Institute Leeds

APPENDIX TWO

Assessing Allowances for Holiday, Sickness and Study Leave

Percentage allowances added to hospital staffing figures

Once the in-post staffing needs have been calculated, a further allowance should be added which reflects holiday, sickness and study leave requirements.

Some services may have agreed allowances, others may be changing their allowances as Trust Boards renegotiate holiday allowances.

The following examples are intended to enable managers to calculate and analyse whatever allowance is given.

In the example given in the text, a basic allowance of 17.3 per cent has been added. This reflects a minimum allowance of:

- 5 weeks annual leave plus 10 days bank holiday = 7 weeks
- 2 weeks for sickness and a small amount of study leave = minimum of 9 weeks per annum added to in-post figures
- 9 = 17.3 per cent of a year (9/52 = 0.173 x 100 = 17.3 per cent).

If three weeks are assessed to allow for sickness/study leave = 10 weeks/52 = 19.2 per cent.

If four weeks are assessed to allow for sickness/study leave = 11 weeks/52 = 21.15 per cent.

By the same token, 12 weeks = 23.08 per cent, 13 weeks = 25 per cent.

Community caseload/hospital and community combined work

Calculation of annual hours per midwife and holiday/sickness and study leave allowances

As before, if allowances are based on current holiday allowances plus a minimum of two weeks sickness and study leave.

52 weeks per annum:

- Deduct: 7 weeks holiday = 5 weeks annual leave plus 10 bank holidays
- Deduct: a *minimum* allowance of 2 weeks sickness and/or study leave
- Total: 9 weeks (= 17.3 per cent of total 52 weeks).

52 - 9 = 43 weeks x 37.5 hours per week = 1612.5 hours per annum per w.t.e. midwife. This would reflect *total establishment needs.*

Based on agreed local terms and sickness rates

In many units different rates apply. If this is the case in a local situation, then the local allowance should be used to calculate annual hours e.g.

- 3 weeks sickness plus holidays = 52 - 10 weeks = 42 x 37.5 = 1575 midwife hours per annum (19.2 per cent allowance)

- 4 weeks sickness plus holidays = 52 - 10 weeks = 41 x 37.5 = 1537.5 midwife hours per annum (21.2 per cent allowance)

- 5 weeks sickness plus holidays = 52 -12 weeks = 40 x 37.5 = 1500 midwife hours per annum (23.0 per cent allowance).

Formula for Calculating Caseload Midwife Hours per Case and Traditional Community Midwife Hours per Case

Formula for assessing midwife hours per client for caseload based work (hospital or home delivery)

Antenatal care

- Booking visit/initial planning etc. = 1.5 hours
- Ultrasound = 0.5 hour
- Antenatal contacts at 26, 34, 36, 38, 40 weeks = 5 hours
- Parentcraft, hospital visits for client and partner = 2.0 hours
- Total = *9* hours

Intrapartum care

Includes labour, delivery and follow-up visit or discharge from hospital within six hours (includes some allowance for a second midwife to attend a home delivery)

- Total = *17* hours

Postnatal care

Includes visits at hospital or home:

1. Low risk/normal outcomes - transferred from hospital on 1st to 3rd day postnatal and discharged around 10th -12th day, 12 visits are needed = *10* hours

2. Complicated cases needing longer postnatal care in hospital, transferred 4-7 days, discharge around 15th - 18th postnatal day = *15* hours.

Total hours per case

- Normal/low risk: 36 hours per case + 5 per cent admin/management = *38* hours
- Complicated /high risk: 41 hours per case + 5 per cent admin/management = *43* hours.

Administration allowances

The hours per case given in the two formulae include all the direct and indirect care i.e. paper work, telephone contacts etc. for each client. Study leave is included in the staffing hours per annum. Administration allowances of five per cent for team/group meetings and liaison which are additional to contacts related to client care, plus meetings with managers, audit etc. (5 per cent = 2 hours per case over and above client related administration).

Travel allowances also need to be added (see Appendix 4).

Formula for assessing midwife hours for traditional care of clients delivered by hospital staff

Antenatal care (all cases)

Assuming that the midwife is involved in shared antenatal care with GP and hospital, but does not act as lead professional.

*   6.5 hours + 5 per cent administration etc. = 7 hours per case

Postnatal care

1. Low risk: early transfer home: days 1-3 discharged by midwife around days 10/12 = 5 per cent administration etc. = 8.5 + 5 per cent = *9* hours per case

2. High risk/complicated: home 4-7 days, discharged by midwife around day 13-16 = 7 + 5 per cent = *7.5* hours per case.

*   Total hours = low risk = *16* hours
*   High risk, complicated cases: *14.5* hours

(complicated cases need less time because the midwife does not visit in hospital as the caseload based midwife would).

Administration allowances

The hours per case given in the two formulae include all the direct and indirect care i.e. paper work, telephone contacts etc. for each client. Study leave is included in the staffing hours per annum. Administration allowances of five per cent account for team/group meetings and liaison which are additional to contacts related to client care, plus meetings with managers, audit etc. (five per cent = two hours per case over and above client related administration).

Travel allowances also need to be added (see Appendix 4).

APPENDIX FOUR

Rationale for Travel Allowances in Different Locations

There seems to be a dearth of information on the amount of midwife time spent travelling around and between clients homes, the hospital, community services etc. Where local data are available via Korner or other audit procedures then that is the travel allowance which should be added to the midwife hours required.

Where such data are not available the following recommendations may be of help to managers.

Travel allowances and working locations

• Ten per cent: mainly urban, not heavily congested, small radius for clients within ten miles of bases (3.8 hours for each normal case)

• 15 per cent: mainly urban, with some rural, covering a wider radius of up to 15 mile radius of base (5.7 hours for each normal case)

• 17.5 per cent: either heavily congested urban area (e.g. central areas of main cities) or mixed urban and rural area with radius of up to 20 miles from base (6.65 hours for each normal case)

• 20 per cent: mainly rural, longer distance into main unit, radius of 20 - 40 miles for caseload midwives (7.6 hours for each normal case).

Allowances above 20 per cent should be verified by local data and are likely to be needed in rural areas with limited road systems e.g. North of Scotland, Lake District, parts of East Anglia.

APPENDIX FIVE

Assessing Midwife Hours per Annum

In many situations, it is preferable to calculate midwife hours per annum to calculate annual hours per whole time equivalent.

1. On current holiday allowances plus *minimum* of 2 weeks sickness and study leave, annual hours per w.t.e. are equal to:

    52 weeks per annum
    deduct 5 weeks leave and 10 bank holidays and a further 2 weeks for sickness and study leave = 9 weeks.

    52 - 9 = 43 working weeks x 37.5 hours per week = 1612.5 annual hours per w.t.e. midwife (= 17.3 per cent allowance).

2. Based on different allowances:
    3 weeks sickness and study leave and holidays = 52 - 10 weeks
    = 42 weeks x 37.5 hours
    = 1575 annual hours per w.t.e. midwife (=19.2 per cent allowance).

    4 weeks sickness and study leave and holidays = 52 -11 weeks
    = 41 weeks x 37.5 hours
    = 1537.5 annual hours per w.t.e. midwife (=21.2 per cent allowance).

Index

A

activity analysis 12, 18, 87
allowances for administration and management 42, 86, 90, 92, 93, 103, 106, 116-118, 170
annual hours per midwife 90, 91, 116, 118, 124-131, 136, 146, 168, 172
antenatal care
  community 112, 114, 116-118
  hospital 78-81, 84
    93, 102, 117, 118
antenatal cases on delivery suites 15, 73
antenatal clinics
    19, 104, 109, 126, 134, 135
apgar score 23, 24, 27, 32
Audit commission 7, 18, 46
Auld, M. 3, 4

B

Ball, J.A. 2, 4, 5, 11, 17, 22, 24, 66
Ball, J.A., Goldstone, L.A. et al. 4
Ball, J.A., Washbrook, M. 22
Ball J.A. et al. 4, 5, 8, 18, 46, 99, 115, 116, 125
Ball, J.A., Hurst, K. 7
Ball, J.A., Oreschnik, R.W. 7
Barr, et al. 3, 4
bed days per category 76, 78, 79
bed occupancy
    12, 71, 73, 76, 78, 80, 83
beds required 69-84
Bell, A., Storey, C. 4

Birthrate data produced:
  daily mean no of cases 37, 41, 72-74, 147
  midwife time per category 14, 17, 22, 29-35, 37, 40, 43, 71-72 147, 148, 150
  workload ratios and indices 40, 41, 44, 48-64, 147, 151
Birthrate data used for:
  assessing beds needed 71-84
  intrapartum staffing 39-64, 140, 142, 146, 147, 150
  managing change 144, 145, 146, 147, 152
  planning community workloads 120-122
  staffing wards 85-110
Birthrate score system 20-64
  principles 22-25
  instructions for score system 26-28
    case-studies 31-35
    categories X, A and R 15, 23, 28, 36
    delivered cases: categories I-V 20-36
    escort duties 30, 42
    flying squad 30, 42, 45
    length of time in delivery suite 23, 28-35,
    multiple births 24, 27, 33
    validity and reliability checks 36, 38
    score sheet 23, 24, 31, 166
    setting up the system 36-38
    theatre cases 30, 42
Birthrate system: development 10-19
  clinical indicators 5, 14, 15, 18
  data produced 16, 36, 39, 43, 47, 65
  infants score 15, 26, 33
  principles 11, 14-17, 23, 36
  reliability 17, 36
  score system and categories 15-16, 18, 23-24, 26-28, 35
  validity 17
breech deliveries 13